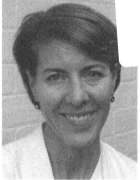

Nicola Gates PhD is a clinical neuropsychologist with more than twenty-five years' experience working with adults to improve their brain health, cognitive function and mental wellbeing. She is the bestselling author of *A Brain for Life*, based on her academic research investigating the prevention of dementia. In her clinical practice, Brain and Mind Psychology, Nicola combines neuropsychology and mindfulness with positive psychology to improve individual's lives. To enrich her own life, Nicola has a fifty-acre property where she keeps bees and is establishing a large native garden.

www.brainandmindpsychology.com

THE FEEL GOOD GUIDE TO
MENOPAUSE

Dr Nicola Gates

ABC
BOOKS

All personal recounts are written by the women involved
and have been lightly edited only.

This book is within the self-help genre and is not designed to provide
definitive or individual advice, and is not a substitute for appropriate care
from a registered medical or health professional.

 The ABC 'Wave' device is a trademark of the
Australian Broadcasting Corporation and is used
under licence by HarperCollins*Publishers* Australia.

First published in Australia in 2019
by HarperCollins*Publishers* Australia Pty Limited
ABN 36 009 913 517
harpercollins.com.au

HarperCollins*Publishers*
Level 13, 201 Elizabeth Street, Sydney, NSW 2000, Australia
Unit D1, 63 Apollo Drive, Rosedale, Auckland 0632, New Zealand
A 53, Sector 57, Noida, UP, India
1 London Bridge Street, London, SE1 9GF, United Kingdom
Bay Adelaide Centre, East Tower, 22 Adelaide Street West, 41st Floor,
 Toronto, Ontario, M5H 4E3, Canada
195 Broadway, New York, NY 10007

A catalogue record for this book is available from the National Library of Australia

ISBN 978 0 7333 3874 8 (paperback)
ISBN 978 1 4607 0903 0 (ebook)

Cover design by Hazel Lam, HarperCollins Design Studio
Cover image by Ruth Black / Stocksy.com / 995121
Typeset in Sabon LT Std by Kelli Lonergan
Printed and bound in Australia by McPherson's Printing Group
The papers used by HarperCollins in the manufacture of this book are natural,
recyclable product made from wood grown in sustainable plantation forests.
The fibre source and manufacturing processes meet recognised international
environmental standards, and carry certification.

I dedicate this book to my darling, supportive and accommodating husband, Simon. I love and appreciate your constancy and commitment. I thrive because you support me to be who I am and adore me always.

Contents

Introduction

Menopause is, like puberty, a time of massive hormonal change, but in the opposite direction as our bodies shift from being fertile to infertile. This transition is a significant time of change in women's lives, and like all change it can be challenging. Whether menopause is overall a negative and overwhelming time or one of net growth and transformation depends not only on the severity of our symptoms, but also our knowledge, attitude and self-compassion, the support we can access and our capacity to blossom into the third stage of our lives.

We know menopause will happen and we have some idea what to expect, but the dawning realisation that subtle signs indicate that we are in the menopause transition can still take us by surprise. Our well-known bodies start to function differently and can feel foreign. The first noticeable symptoms that things are changing are likely to be different and irregular periods, perhaps hot flushes, or maybe disturbed sleep. We are familiar with these visible physical symptoms and can anticipate them. We keep vigilant, check in with ourselves, and perhaps start investigating treatment options. But what happens when we experience unexpected changes, less familiar from popular culture, or which are invisible? We are thrown off kilter, and don't know what is happening or how to manage.

Although women make up half the world's population there is limited awareness and understanding about how menopause affects our thinking and emotions. While we have the knowledge to put women in outer space we still do not have enough knowledge about how our hormones impact our inner space – our brains and minds.

Our brains and reproductive organs have been intimately connected since our conception and have been talking to each other ever since through a complex communication and feedback system. Our female sex hormones do a lot more than give us periods each month. They have major roles in our general health maintenance, thinking and behaviour. Too often women and their treating health professionals do not recognise the susceptibility of the brain and mind to hormone fluctuations and these symptoms are ignored or misdiagnosed. But that need not be the case.

As a clinical neuropsychologist I am particularly interested in the brain–mind–behaviour relationship and am fascinated by how the fluctuations in hormone levels change the way our brain operates and how we think and feel. The fluctuations in, and ultimate loss of, hormones impact brain structures, brain chemistry, cognitive functions such as memory, as well as mood, emotion, stress levels and behaviour.

In my clinical practice I notice more women in their mid-forties to early fifties coming in with concerns for their memory and 'brain fog', and others with anxiety, stress and depression. Some women who have mothers with dementia are specifically fearful they too might have early dementia. They report that their brains are like sieves as they cannot hold on to information and forget conversations, tasks, words and names, or have other cognitive issues such as indecision, poor attention and slowed thinking. There is another group whose primary concerns are feelings of emotional disconnection, who have a sense of being easily overwhelmed and stressed or feel increased anxiety and depression. They are unsettled, concerned and bewildered about what is happening within them.

The lack of awareness of these less obvious brain and mind menopausal changes can make the transition experience unnecessarily difficult, reduce the likelihood of compassionate support, and limit intervention.

As I began to write this book my own life unfolded unpredictably, as life is wont to do, and in such a way that I personally needed to update my knowledge of menopause. I was sitting opposite my doctor discussing what I had thought were normal peri-menopause symptoms when she said, 'time to put it in a bucket'. She was referring to my uterus. My unpredictable yet heavy periods were not normal at all. I felt some sadness at losing my wonderful womb, which symbolised motherhood for me – it had after all been the temporary home for my two children – but also considerable relief. In among that emotional mix I had to get my head around the possibility of waking post-operatively without my ovaries and in menopause. Whether I would have a *natural* menopause, or an abrupt *medical* menopause, would be determined during surgery.

My ovaries were 'beautiful', the surgeon said, so they had remained. I thought I would continue through natural menopause. Except, in another left-hand turn I was subsequently diagnosed with grade-3 invasive breast cancer. It was oestrogen and progesterone driven. My ovaries may have been beautiful, but they were too prolific for my age. After a double mastectomy (which I pragmatically embraced to be cancer-free), my ovaries needed to be immediately decommissioned prior to commencing anti-cancer medication. I went into a very sudden medically induced menopause.

In the wake of this treatment as I investigated the brain fog of my menopause, it became clear to me in a very direct way that the role of oestrogen in the brain and mind has been terribly underestimated. In fact it is largely an untold story.

Research has only really started in the past decade, and the lag of ten to twenty years between medical research and medical practice means there is limited public awareness and understanding of the impact of hormones and hormonal changes on women's brains and minds. I want to close this gap in information for women and share the science story of menopause from a neuropsychological perspective. Knowledge allows us to identify our key concerns to target and increases our management options. We do need to take a broad view beyond hormone therapies as lifestyle and mindstyle strategies contribute so much to our overall health and wellbeing through the transition, abrupt or natural. One thing I can confirm is attitude profoundly impacts how we experience menopause and life. All changes we make are likely to have a wonderful positive domino effect onto other symptoms and all areas of our lives now and in the future.

There are five key messages in this book.

- First, that the brain changes during the transition as it adapts to a different, less potent form of oestrogen, but it *does* adapt.
- Second, that there can be an impact on mental health, but that doesn't mean these changes are permanent or indicate a mental illness.
- Third, that a positive attitude and a proactive approach will make a profound difference to your menopause experience. The adoption of a healthy lifestyle and an optimistic mindstyle will help you thrive.
- Fourth, and this is a caution, menopause is a big change, but it might not be the cause of all your difficulties. There are multiple other factors in play that are related to age, life stage, relationship status and environment that may be unhelpful and there may be something else in your life that needs to change.
- Lastly, the guarantee. Menopause will liberate you from cycling sex hormones and herald the start of your third life. The objective here is to ensure that life is a good one.

To illustrate these points, I've included women's stories throughout. These highlight our diverse experiences and give voice to many of our shared difficulties. The stories, for which I am forever grateful, will, I hope, help make the science real and relatable for you.

Skipping through the information on menopause and going straight to management is very tempting, especially if you are feeling desperate to alleviate symptoms. But this may deny you a comprehensive understanding of the journey and ultimately restrict your management options or capacity to identify the best solution/s. Complex overlapping processes that generate multiple changes for body, brain and mind often need complex solutions. It is important to understand all that is happening and how things are related.

I've drawn on cutting-edge research to pack this book with information: I want to demystify menopause as well as give you practical ways to manage symptoms and improve your quality of life. The complicated medical research is distilled into science bites. The self-care summaries provide plenty of options, so you can make informed choices to manage this significant body–brain–mind transition. This book is about optimistic empowerment with information and strategies so that the menopause transition becomes a time of transformation. Now is the time for you to truly flourish.

HER-STORY

Women have profoundly different health lives from men. Our female health story is largely dictated by our sexual reproductive hormones – which direct our sexual development through puberty, support menstrual cycles and pregnancy, and ultimately leave us during menopause. They also impact our entire wellbeing, influencing physical and mental health. However, until recently our biology has often been confused with other forces.

Ancient and patriarchal beliefs about women and their bodies have significantly influenced medical practice for generations, and account for the lack of information and research on the health journey of women. The menopause transition is only one part of the bigger tapestry of women's unique health. To nurture and cherish our female bodies and confirm our access to appropriate medical diagnoses and treatment we need to understand menopause in this broader context of medical practice in the past as it still impacts today.

Women's health and access to services has continually been complicated by prejudice, and theological and socio-political influences. Women bear new life, a truly remarkable capacity; however, rather than being celebrated women's reproductive bodies have largely been viewed pejoratively. Women were believed to be inferior to men, physically, mentally, emotionally and spiritually, and 'femaleness' has been seen as a weakness and a curse, and significantly misunderstood.

The leadership of state and religion *and* the practice of medicine were dominated by men and, as men do not have periods, pregnancies or menopause, their lack of experiential knowledge, coupled with prejudice, has had a huge impact on the diagnosis and treatment of women's health issues for centuries.

Hysteria

The first word we know of being given to singularly female health issues was 'hysteria', from the Greek word *hysterika*, meaning womb (uterus). It is believed the term was first used in ancient Egypt and then in a gynaecological text in the fifth century BC by Hippocrates. It referred to the 'wandering womb', as the uterus was believed to be free floating within the body and its movement the cause of women's disorders. The uterus was prone to 'get sick', especially if deprived of sex and pregnancy, which acted to tie the organ in place. The direction in which the womb wandered was believed to explain the diversity of symptoms and complaints reported by women.

The next major influence on women's health was Christianity. Through the prism of Christian theology, women's health issues were perceived as 'the curse of Eve' and therefore could be justifiably ignored. When biblical Eve took a bite of the apple and offered it to Adam, and he chose to eat it, Eve was held responsible for their expulsion from the Garden of Eden and for the sinful downfall of humans. Pain during childbirth and menstruation, and presumably menopausal discomfort, were seen by early physicians as God's well-earned punishment of women and a constant reminder of Eve's error. As a result, there was no significant push to address the unique health issues women face. They were simply a woman's lot in life.

In the seventeenth century Descartes had a major impact upon western medicine as he demonstrated that actions previously ascribed to the soul were due to the body's organs and brain, and by the eighteenth century, symptoms of hysteria were linked to the brain rather than the uterus. Thankfully, because in severe cases of hysteria women underwent hysterectomies to remove the uterus to cure them.

The conflation of physical/sexual reproductive and psychological symptoms, however, continued.

Hysteria became an exceedingly common diagnosis of female psychological disorder or 'nervousness'. The understanding was that 'excessive emotional reactivity' was converted into multiple and diverse symptoms including faintness, nervousness, irritability and non-compliant behaviour along with the more physical ones of fluid retention, shortness of breath and loss of appetite. Many female concerns were therefore dismissed as heightened 'emotionality' rather than being legitimate medical or health issues.

By the twentieth century the diagnosis of hysteria was in decline for two primary reasons. First, the number of symptoms ascribed to hysteria were so broad and could be applied to so many recognised medical conditions that it was no longer helpful. Second, the development of medical investigative and scientific procedures enabled the identification of more specific physical and psychiatric conditions.

Freud reclassified many of the symptoms linked to hysteria into a new set of diagnoses called 'female neuroses'. This female-specific set of disorders remained in diagnostic manuals until 1980 when it was replaced with the non-sex-specific term 'hysterical neurosis'. Diagnostic terms have continually been superseded and the latest is 'functional neurological disorder' (FND), which represents the crossover between neurological, physical and psychiatric symptoms, and is largely applied to women.

Medical symptoms reported by women continue to be arbitrarily attributed to their emotionality rather than to a medical health issue. For example, I had a client who felt 'not quite right' and excessively tired after completing a major work project and was told by her treating doctor that it was stress, she had 'over-exerted' herself and needed to see a psychologist. I might work in brain and mental health, but I do not make assumptions. I suggested she have blood tests to exclude an underlying health issue. She called me a week later to say thanks. The blood tests revealed an elevated white cell count: she had breast cancer.

Medical bias

Women outnumber and outlive men. Women also use more health and medical services than men. Yet there is a significant disconnection between women's health, longevity and their use of medical services, and the amount of female-oriented medical research. This is because until recently women have not been involved in, or the subject of, medicine. The lack of women in medical science has had far-reaching implications for women's health and wellbeing. For example, menstrual cramps (dysmenorrhoea) were considered psychological or psychosomatic complaints right up to the 1940s. The lack of scientific knowledge regarding the female body and hormones meant there was no medical evidence to contradict the psychiatric interpretation with a biological explanation.

The United Nations states that health equality is necessary for gender equality so understanding female hormones and improving women's health is crucial. However, most medical research, including that into alternative and complementary therapies, has involved men to the exclusion of women: men perform the research and are also the subject of that research. Until very recently it was rare for women to practice medicine or to be involved in medical research. Less well known has been the lack of female animals in experimental research, and the failure of medical research to include women in clinical and treatment trials. Although women take more medication than men, until recently drug or pharmacological research and clinical trials have predominantly been conducted on men only. For example, in the initial studies of aspirin in preventing heart attacks in the UK, over twenty-two thousand men were studied. No women were included at all. Consequently, when the research results were extrapolated, and treatment recommendations applied to women, they were wrong. It is now understood that low-dose aspirin has different beneficial effects in women than it does in men because of the positive influence of our sex hormones. Given we now understand oestrogen has a protective role in cardiovascular health – and that women in child-bearing years produce significantly more oestrogen than men – the absence of women in heart studies has been a notable oversight. There are recognised sex differences in the effect of medication, but we still do not understand if there are possible differences in the effect of aspirin on women's cardiovascular health across their reproductive stage, including pre-, peri- and post-menopause. The exclusion of women from clinical research is bad for women's health and does not help medical science progress either, especially in terms of developing oestrogen-based treatments for diseases such as dementia.

Guidelines directing researchers to include women were not mandated in most countries until the 1990s. One of the most common reasons given for the exclusion of women from medical research is that our hormonal changes, during our fertile years and menopause, complicate research! As a result, research continues to neglect the effect that a woman's reproductive status may have on medication and treatment.

As mentioned earlier, medical research has also been biased in that traditionally only male animals have been included in cell and preclinical research. These trials are used to guide human clinical trials, and the absence of female animals helps in part to explain why the findings from cellular and bio-medical studies are not replicated in trials using women.

Ideology has also influenced research. For example, in the 1990s it was suggested by the first female tenured medical scientist at Harvard, Professor Ruth Hubbard, that there was great overlap between men and women in 'all traits except those directly involved with procreation'. At that time some medical research was influenced by the socio-political need to prove there were no differences between men and women to ensure equality. This belief has limited the understanding of how sex hormones impact health.

We are now developing an understanding of hormones and how the sexual reproductive hormones significantly influence brain development and contribute to the physiological, emotional and behavioural differences seen between men and women. As a result, there is now recognition that sex-specific health and sex-specific treatment are crucial to maximise individual health and wellbeing.

Science bite: What are hormones?

Hormones are chemical messengers in the body and were discovered in the early twentieth century. They are made in endocrine glands. The brain signals their release and they travel in the bloodstream to their target receptor tissues and organs. They are involved in growth, metabolism, brain function and reproduction, as well as mood and behaviour. Sex hormones are those responsible for sexual reproduction. In women, the significant sex hormones are oestrogen and progesterone, and were first isolated in 1939. See Part 2 Hormone Health for more.

Medicine and menopause

In addition to medical biases there are more excuses as to why medical research specifically into menopause has been so patchy to date. First, symptoms vary between women, they can change in frequency, intensity and duration, and whether the menopause was natural or medical makes a significant difference to the experience and the risks for other health conditions. Second, many symptoms are not linked just to menopause but are also associated with increasing age and other medical conditions. Third, the age that we start having periods (menarche) and then the age we stop having them due to menopause has also been found to have different health consequences for women in later life. Lastly, as a result of differences in our genes, environment, life experiences, lifestyle and mindstyle, we become more unique with age.

These factors make research difficult to navigate, but not impossible. Significant funding is necessary, along with medical curiosity and rigour. For example, research into coronary heart disease in post-menopausal women, their biggest killer, remains inconclusive because of a lack of well-designed studies. In contrast, well-funded research into alcohol-related cancer, which shares similar confounds of age, hormones, lifestyle and genes, along with frequency, amount and duration of alcohol consumption, has established that the consumption of fifty or more grams of alcohol per day leads to two to three times greater risk of developing alcohol-related cancers than not drinking. Alcohol is a lifestyle choice, and excessive alcohol intake concerns a minority of individuals, predominantly men. It's ridiculous that this even needs to be said, but more money and interest in women's health could considerably improve the quality and sophistication of research, and provide health recommendations to improve cardiovascular health in post-menopausal women.

15

Most of the available information regarding menopause concerns the number and frequency of menopause symptoms. This research is not particularly helpful because the frequency rates of given symptoms are often no better than chance, and because the studies are often poor quality. Nevertheless, they form the foundation for information upon which health professionals and women rely.

Identifying symptoms does not isolate cause and effect, which is necessary to determine the best treatment strategies and develop suitable management options. The limited research, along with a lack of comprehensive understanding of symptoms, has implications for investigations into the risks for diseases associated with oestrogen loss, such as the abovementioned cardiovascular disease, along with diabetes mellitus, osteoporosis and the number-two killer of women, dementia. Understanding the relationships between lifetime exposure to endogenous oestrogen (which women make within their bodies), the intake of exogenous oestrogens (from external sources such as hormone therapies and the environment) and possible health risks may lead to more effective prevention and management.

Things are changing. Women are now present in all areas of medicine – as treating health professionals and in research, training and leadership positions. In many countries there has been a positive shift to specifically investigate women's health issues and to identify the best forms of treatment for women. Western medicine is also on the verge of practising individualised medicine, which will not only consider sex but also individual characteristics including genes, hormones and history. Therefore, awareness and acceptance of female hormonal differences in body, brain and mind represent a crucial step towards improved and individualised health care. My hope is that medical and health practices will change rapidly now and that our female reproductive lives become integrated into our health care.

Being female

Menopause may concern both women and men, but it only occurs in those born biologically female. Our sex hormones are different from male sex hormones, so our bodies, brains, emotions and behaviour are also different. We have a lot in common with men but the differences between us are significant and the biological evidence is concrete.

All human embryos start to develop the same, then sexual differentiation appears according to our sex chromosomes. In women our XX chromosomes dictate that the gonads carry on developing into ovaries. In men, the XY chromosomes change the development path so that the gonads become testes and the pattern of masculinisation begins.

Once the ovaries have developed, our primary and secondary sex characteristics are determined according to gene instruction and the sex hormones produced at specific points in development. Our female sex hormones trigger an incredible cascade of biological and physiological changes that give rise to a woman's reproductive potential, including female anatomy and brain, and influence our mind/psychology and behaviour.

Biological sex is not the same as gender, which is largely how people identify themselves. Gender is not biological but a human construct that reflects cultural expectations and personal and societal perceptions of one's sex. In this book we are talking about female biological sex at birth, not gender identity as a woman. If you have ovaries, or have had ovaries, this book applies to you, because you were born female.

Females and males share the same sex hormones, we just make them in different places and in different amounts. The ovaries produce oestrogen, progesterone and a small amount of testosterone; in men testosterone is produced in their testes in large quantities along with a little oestrogen. Although we are all on a continuum, females and males are most different during their sexual reproductive years when their sex hormone levels are high, and then the differences begin to wane with increasing age. A post-menopausal woman for example will end up with about as much oestrogen as a man of similar age.

Our reproductive bodies

In order to better understand the profound changes we experience during the menopausal transition it is necessary to revisit what our female reproductive hormones do across our lifespan. Once our ovaries are present, our development is influenced by our sex hormones. Oestrogen is the primary sex hormone that we think of that makes us female, and is the same as estrogen: these are simply different spellings depending upon where you live. For simplicity, we will stick to oestrogen. There are three different forms of oestrogen in women, depending on reproductive stage. The other major sex hormones made in the ovaries are progesterone and a small amount of testosterone, which is classed as an androgen. Two additional hormones also responsible for our reproductive health are follicle stimulating hormone (FSH) and luteinising hormone (LH) produced in the brain's pituitary gland.

Science bite: The three oestrogens

Oestrogens are predominantly secreted by the ovaries and are synthesised from cholesterol, with the amounts we produce varying over the course of our reproductive cycle and reproductive life.

Oestrone (E_1) is the main source of oestrogen before puberty and after menopause and it is the 'weakest' form of oestrogen. The ovaries produce only a little oestrone, while most oestrone is produced by adipose tissue (fat tissue) from the conversion of

---

androstenedione from the adrenal glands. Too much stress reduces the production of androstenedione as the adrenals are too busy making stress hormones. Being too thin can also be a problem as there may not be enough fatty tissue to produce oestrone.

Oestradiol (E$_2$) is the most active form of oestrogen. It supports reproduction and is produced during our fertile years and is the most potent and most common form of oestrogen. Oestradiol is produced in the ovarian granulosa cells which line the follicles of the ovaries. Follicles contain eggs and as they mature the size and number of the granulosa cells increase, which progressively raises the level of oestrogen. It is produced in puberty for the development of secondary sex characteristics and fertility (menses), and it's active for psychological and physical functions throughout adulthood before menopause.

Oestriol (E$_3$) is often only thought of as the pregnancy oestrogen, as it is produced in the placenta from around eight weeks' gestation. Oestriol increases steadily in pregnancy as it is made from a chemical that the developing baby produces in its adrenal gland, and surges three weeks before birth. It also exists in very low levels normally in non-pregnant women.

Immediately after we are born, our oestrogen levels are very high and stay high from one to twenty-four months of age as we continue to grow and develop according to our sex. Surprisingly, there is very limited research on post-natal sex hormone production and the development of sex-specific biology and behaviour. Our oestrogen levels then quieten down and appear relatively stable until late childhood when the brain's hypothalamus tells our body it is time to complete our growth and development for sexual reproduction. Our sex hormones increase again and we enter puberty.

Once in puberty, we gain extra weight, and this natural weight gain supports oestrogen production as well as becoming an important store of energy throughout womanhood to support potential pregnancies. It also provides protection for maintaining the health of the inner organs and uterus. Keep in mind that oestrogen is produced from fat deposits as well as the ovaries, and that we need to be an appropriate weight for all hormone health, including fertility, pregnancy and getting through menopause.

During puberty, we also undergo tissue growth and cell proliferation in specific areas in the body to develop our secondary sex characteristics of breasts and hips, as well as the maturation of the uterus for menstruation and ultimately pregnancy. Our vaginal walls thicken, and vaginal secretion begins, which is protective as well as lubricating. Gradually, our sexual reproductive hormones get to sufficient levels to support menses and our periods start, and we have an increase in testosterone to stimulate sex drive.

Oestrogen prepares our bodies for ovulation and sex. Our ovaries do not make eggs – we are born with all our eggs present – but hormones stimulate the maturation and release of egg/s, termed ovulation, along with the secretion of oestrogen. It is the gradual loss of our eggs that leads to the loss of oestrogen and, ultimately, we have no more viable eggs and are in menopause.

The menstrual cycle is broken into two phases: pre- and post-ovulation. The pre-ovulation phase, or follicular phase, is when eggs mature. At the beginning of this phase the pituitary gland in our brain sends out the follicle stimulating hormone (FSH) and luteinising hormone (LH). Between ten and thirty follicles, which are cells containing immature eggs, begin to ripen and stimulate the ovaries to produce oestrogen.

When the oestrogen levels in the bloodstream are at their highest the hypothalamus in the brain sends hormones to instruct the follicle/s to release the matured egg/s. Usually only one egg has developed to full maturity and the others break down and are reabsorbed by the body. During this phase oestrogen changes the vaginal and cervical mucus and internal environment to be more sperm friendly and stimulates the growth of the uterine lining, causing it to thicken. This makes the body ready for sexual intercourse and for a potentially fertilised egg.

Have you ever noticed that you may have higher libido at certain times in your cycle? Studies suggest that women do tend to have more sexual thoughts and are more likely to engage in sexual activity right before ovulation. Testosterone helps to regulate our energy, mental state and importantly our sex drive (libido), and like oestrogen it goes up pre-ovulation, and down during the menopausal transition.

Progesterone, the other important hormone produced by the ovaries, is produced during the luteal phase or the second half of the menstrual cycle, post-ovulation, when the egg is released. This phase is all about preparing the body for possible conception and promoting pregnancy and the survival of the foetus. Progesterone encourages the growth of milk-producing glands in the breast, which explains why many women get tender and enlarged breasts ahead of their period. It also has a calming effect on our mood and acts as an anti-depressant, which is necessary to support pregnancy.

When we do not become pregnant the whole cycle shuts down, with oestrogen and progesterone levels dropping. This leads to the breakdown of the endometrium and we experience a period. The period is the discharge of blood, cells and mucus that formed the uterine lining. Generally, women will lose about 50 to 100 millilitres of fluid with each period, though this varies between cycles and women. If your periods are heavy or unusual (for you), check with your medical practitioner. Do not assume or think that your periods are changing simply because you may be in peri-menopause; there are other medical conditions that impact periods such as hormonal disorders, anorexia, fibroids, endometriosis and cancer.

The transition through puberty to sexual reproductive maturity takes between two and five years. For most girls, menses starts somewhere between age ten and fifteen – with twelve being the average age – and it matters for the rest of your life. We have reached maturity when our oestrogen, progesterone and testosterone fluctuate in a monthly pattern and we have a regular menstrual cycle. We have also adapted to the surges in our hormones, learned to cope with our periods, and got to know our fertile bodies.

In the background to the primary role in our sexual reproductive lives, our sex hormones are quietly maintaining our general body health. For example, oestrogen is supporting bone density, the health of the heart and vascular system, controlling electrolyte balance to support the body's largest organ, the skin, and much much more.

Science bite: Wonderful eggs

Biological females are born with all their potential eggs, between one and two million of them. This is important to understand because the health of our grandmothers has a big impact upon our health, including that of our eggs. The potential eggs that became us were made in our mothers' ovaries when they were foetuses in utero! The number and quality of eggs steadily decreases, so by puberty the number of potential ova has dropped to between 300,000 and 400,000, and then from the mid-thirties there is a steep decline.

There are about fifteen to twenty ova enclosed in each follicle. Over the course of the reproductive lifespan approximately three hundred to four hundred ova will mature to ovulation. The ovarian gran cells respond to follicle development and secrete oestrogen. One follicle becomes dominant and suppresses the development

---

of the other follicles, which then die, and the dominant follicle is supported to mature. With each cycle, up to a thousand follicles will be lost for good. As oestrogen begins to rise it switches off the production of FSH, otherwise we would continue to lose follicles, so the system is finely tuned.

The ovulatory phase begins with an increase in LH to trigger the follicle to release the ova from the ovary. The tiny ova are about the size of a full stop on this page and are visible to the naked eye. However, compared to other cells in the body they are rather large, and are sixteen times larger than sperm. They have about twelve to twenty-four hours to get fertilised. That gorgeous egg influences which sperm will fertilise it − with a selective preference for sperm with intact DNA − by releasing a compound to soften the outer layer, allowing only the specific selected sperm to enter.

The female brain

Oestrogen supports the body's fundamental organ – the brain. The brain regulates and controls hundreds of different bodily functions and organs such as our heart and stomach as well as governing our thoughts, emotions and behaviour. It does all these things through two communication systems using neurotransmitters and hormones. Oestrogen is crucial to many of these brain–body and body–brain functions, with the brains of both women and men having oestrogen and oestrogen receptors. They also both have progesterone, but very little is known at present about progesterone in the brain. Although women and men share the same sex hormones, when brain development, cognitive processing and genes are examined, there are more than two thousand genes showing differences in expression based on sex, which means our brains are alike but different.

When women feel that menopause is changing their brains and/or influencing their emotions they are right. Oestrogen affects brain development, function and behaviour, and there are critical periods in development when the brain is more sensitive to the influence of sex hormones. It makes sense. Our reproductive bodies are different from men's, so our brain and behaviour need to be different too. The field of neuroendocrinology is devoted to exploring how various hormones change brain chemistry and its structure to dictate certain behaviours. Essentially hormones ensure that behaviour, which is directed by the brain, is consistent with what is happening in the body. A simple example is how oxytocin acts in the brain to both trigger birth and maximise protective and nurturing maternal behaviour once the baby is born and to enhance its survival. The huge range of potential behaviours we may have is genetically determined, however the actual specific behaviours we each develop are influenced by the environment. The process is highly complex with multiple factors influencing the process of feminisation in women, in which a female pattern of brain anatomical and behavioural organisation develops.

Not all brain development is linked to sex hormones. Neuroplastic changes occur in response to learning and experience as well as genetics, environment, health, lifestyle and mindstyle. Our sense of ourselves and our brains is ultimately the product of multiple factors and their relationships. Therefore, we need to be comfortable in understanding our brains (and genders) as existing on a spectrum rather than being binary. But understanding the sex differences in brain physiology and responses to oestrogen is important for understanding the nature and origins of sex-specific healthy stages, medical conditions and psychiatric illnesses, and for designing hormone-based therapies for both women and men.

Differences in sex hormones and androgen and oestrogen receptors within a developing foetus ensure that these brain differences develop. Sex-specific genes are also expressed differently in the brain and so further contribute to brain differences. Neuroanatomical studies reveal that female and male brains have structural differences. The structural, communication and metabolic brain differences between female and male brains translate into cognitive differences too. Cognitive functions such as attention, memory, verbal expression, spatial processing and problem solving are performed differently by women and men although the result is often the same. What is essential to keep in mind is that these differences do not reflect any overall intellectual superiority or advantage to either sex, rather that the brain performs the cognitive tasks differently, as intelligence is equally spread across women and men. We appear to subtly use different parts of the brain to encode memories, sense emotions, recognise faces, solve certain problems and make decisions. We also understand from neuroplasticity that it is not just genes and hormones that influence brain function. There are other factors involved such as exposure and opportunity. Environment (exposure) and experience (opportunity) are crucial. The toys and games that were available, who played them, how play was reinforced, and other stimulating experiences, influence subsequent cognitive capacity. In this way, cognitive function is very dynamic but, notwithstanding those external influential factors, certain patterns of cognitive function are common to women and men.

Interestingly there is now a suggestion that women may also perform cognitive tasks differently depending upon the stage of their menstrual cycle. You may notice within yourself that you are more switched on, dynamic and quick witted at certain times depending upon your cycle – well, it is not in your mind: it's in your hormones!

One area where the differences between female and male brains are widely understood and accepted is mental health. Today there is increasing investigation into the biological reasons (as opposed to the psycho-social-environmental ones) for the sex differences in disease prevalence and age of onset. Schizophrenia is a good example. The disease is equally prevalent in women and men, but age of onset is usually different. In men, onset is early, in the late teens or early twenties. In women, it is mid to late twenties, and then the second peak onset time is after forty-five, coinciding with the menopause transition.

Oestrogen plays a big role in depression and mental health as it appears to reduce psychiatric illnesses: it modulates several neurotransmitters believed to be related to psychoses, such as dopamine, serotonin, noradrenaline and the cholinergic systems. The accepted understanding is that oestrogen exerts an anti-psychotic influence in the brain. Progesterone also impacts mental health as it has a calming anti-anxiety effect. Fluctuating levels of oestrogen and progesterone influence the extent of their protective benefit and the amount of antipsychotic medication that may be required – high levels of these hormones means lower doses of medication. During the menopause transition, women are vulnerable, and the risk of mental illnesses increases as oestrogen and progesterone levels decline. Other menopausal symptoms and life stages may also be problematic.

The brain is an exceedingly dynamic mosaic of structures, functions and experiences that all impact each other. Animal studies examining differences in brain development reveal that prenatal hormones, sex chromosomes, environment and the immune system all have an early role in the development of neural sexual differentiation in women and men, and post-natal differences can continue to arise from specific gene expression, environment and early childcare. Differences in the human brain are therefore the result of a complex mix of all these influences. The important concept here is that female brains are different to men's and menopause changes the brain, how it functions and our behaviour and emotional experiences, and that these changes need to be considered in the management of menopause.

Summary: Protecting your uniqueness

Women and men have different health journeys, different bodies, brains and minds. Make sure your health concerns are heard, that you get the health care you require, and that you feel informed and have options.

- **Find your best fit.** Investigate your own health needs, and review these as they change with age, stage and experience, and develop a care circle of friends and health professionals who fit your beliefs and needs.
- **Celebrate uniqueness and diversity.** With age we become more unique and have more specific needs. Celebrate your individuality and make sure your specific health choices are respected. If you feel different see it as a strength – or perhaps find a tribe, so you keep that sense of belonging. Or make and nurture friendships with those who embrace difference. The balance of variety makes a stronger whole – in our family, community, society and culture. Differences are positive and crucial to our survival.
- **Connect with yourself.** Your body including your brain and thoughts are all interrelated. Your body is your home that carries and protects who you are. Respect and care for your body as it will help you to realise your dreams. Care for the way you talk to yourself, as this conversation impacts your body health, and your sense of who you are.

PART 2

HORMONE HEALTH

Our reproductive journey, including the menopause transition, takes place against the background of our entire endocrine system. It is helpful to understand our hormones broadly before we get to menopause specifics as the transition impacts other hormones, and disruptions in other hormones can significantly impact upon menopause.

The endocrine system is intricate and affects our overall health and wellbeing. It has an impact on things as diverse as sleep, energy, weight and mood. To best support our health and wellbeing during the menopause transition we need to look after our general hormone health as this impacts upon the frequency and intensity of menopause symptoms and influences risk factors for other health conditions.

Our hormones have been changing throughout our entire lives, from conception up until now, and will continue to change as we age. They make up part of the body–brain communication system, along with neurotransmitters, that determines how our body operates, as well as how we think, feel and behave. Hormones have significant and specific roles in supporting our healthy functioning and maintaining homeostasis, and are vital to the whole body. They influence cells, organs and entire body systems – the reproductive system, respiratory system, metabolic system and digestive system, for example – and any disruption or change in our hormones can, therefore, have far-reaching implications for our entire body.

Humans, animals, insects and plants all have hormones governing health and behaviour. Just consider for a moment how you know when you are hungry. The hormone ghrelin gets sent from the stomach to the brain, and you begin to think about food and 'notice' you are hungry and feel motivated to get something to eat, so you do. If you see images of delicious food your brain can similarly respond to motivate you to eat whether you are technically 'hungry' or not.

Hormones are grouped together by type, such as being amino acids, peptides or steroids. The most important types are the peptide hormones, which are small proteins, and steroids, which are lipid (fatty) molecules. The type of hormone determines how each communicates and works. For example, the hormone oxytocin, responsible for our feelings of trust and connection to others, is a peptide hormone. This means it dissolves easily in blood and can be transported widely throughout the body and therefore has many positive benefits, such as making us feel good and boosting our immune systems. But it can't get through fat-rich cell membranes, so it doesn't change body or brain cells.

By comparison, steroid hormones like oestrogen are transported in the bloodstream to their targets and get into cells to tell them what to do. This is important to keep in mind as we go through the menopause journey as oestrogen has a big impact upon lots of organs and cells, including the brain, breasts, heart, blood vessels, uterus, vagina, bladder, liver, bones, skin and gastrointestinal tract. It doesn't just influence organs; it specifically affects emotions and behaviour too. Stop. Reread that list. Oestrogen impacts receptors in all those organs, which explains why we go through such an upheaval when our oestrogen levels change during puberty and the menopause transition.

We all need the same types of hormones to function, but the balance of them may vary between individuals. The amounts of hormones circulating in our blood can also vary in response to the activity of other hormones, our general health, age, attitude, environmental factors and genes.

Science bite: How hormones communicate

Hormone communication is governed by the endocrine system. The endocrine system is made up of a collection of glands and organs: some are in the brain (hypothalamus, pineal gland, pituitary gland) and some are in the body (thyroid, adrenal glands, pancreas, thymus during puberty, gut, testes or ovaries). Endocrine organs produce hormones when activated and then secrete them into the bloodstream so that they are transported throughout the body to work where they are specifically required. The recipients of the hormones are called receptors. Some hormones target specific hormone receptors, some target organs or tissue, and others, like epinephrine (commonly called adrenaline), target nearly every tissue in the body. Some hormones, like triiodothyronine, target nearly every single cell in the body to increase cellular metabolism.

The whole system is regulated by a feedback loop so that when the message is received, and hormones are produced, the recipient site sends a message back to the producer to stop production if there is enough, or to continue to release more hormones if necessary.

Hormone imbalance

Menopause is not a hormonal imbalance; it is a natural change in hormone levels and is a sign of female health. However, when our hormones are not at the ideal levels for our body's requirements we have a hormone imbalance. Hormonal imbalances are not healthy and are due to changes in hormone production and regulation which can cause widespread, serious and life-altering health problems – increased fat storage, weight gain, acne, migraines, loss of libido, fatigue and loss of energy, painful breasts and changes to the menstrual cycle. Some hormone imbalances therefore can present like menopause, for example thyroid disease with its changes to periods, insomnia, hair loss and weight change. Imbalances also complicate menopause, worsening many menopause symptoms, and cause health changes that further increase risks for diseases linked to menopause, such as cardiovascular disease.

Hormone imbalances affect millions of people worldwide every day, and even slight imbalances can lead to fertility changes and increase the risks for some chronic diseases and cancer. The common well-known forms of hormone imbalance are diabetes, thyroid disorders, menstrual irregularities and infertility.

Symptoms of hormone disruption vary depending upon the hormone and its downstream receptor – the target of the hormone message. Common, easily identifiable physical symptoms of hormone imbalance include changes in energy level, appetite and weight, feelings of fatigue, and disturbed sleep. Some symptoms are subtle and less obvious, such as changes in skin moisture, hair loss, increased toileting, bowel and digestive changes, and general aches and pains. Psychological symptoms like feelings of anxiety, stress or sadness may also be experienced. The major health issue is the impact that change in one hormone can have on other hormones. For example, high levels of cortisol from stress impacts insulin which leads to metabolic and appetite changes, and may decrease oestrogen, and heighten menopause symptoms.

Hormonal changes have many potential causes. Some causes are natural – puberty, periods and pregnancy – and some causes can be wonderful – being on holiday or falling in love. However, hormonal disturbances are multi-factorial and not healthy and may include genetic risks, as well as lifestyle factors such as gut health, sleep disturbance, stress, alcohol, over-exercising and environmental toxicity. Because hormones impact multiple body systems, hormone imbalances can cause havoc in many areas of health and wellbeing so they need to be addressed. For many of us, simple lifestyle changes make a positive difference by reducing symptoms, supporting medication benefits and improving quality of life. For others, it may be necessary to use synthetic hormones to effectively treat hormone imbalances: insulin for a person with diabetes; fertility treatments for infertility; and hormone therapy when the ratio of oestrogen to progesterone is not right. Always consult your health practitioner if you have any concerns about your hormone health.

There are dozens of hormones in the body and multiple lifestyle factors that may either support their functions or disrupt them. To best manage menopause, there are four specific areas of hormone disruption discussed here in general hormone health that can impact upon the menopause transition and how well we manage. Our sex hormone health and the other important brain–mind–body hormones, cortisol, serotonin and oxytocin, are discussed in the remaining sections.

Gut–hormone connection

We have recently discovered how important our gut health is to our general health and what impact our food choices have on it. The health of our gut affects our immune system, how much inflammation we have, as well as influencing our mood. Gut health also influences our hormone regulation. In simple brief terms our gut has trillions of micro-organisms, collectively termed the *commensal intestinal microbiome*. The microbiome communicates with our brain and our body via multiple communication systems, including hormones.

There is an amazing triangular relationship between gut health, inflammation and immunity. When our gut community is unhealthy it interacts with our immune system and can cause the release of inflammatory cytokines and stress steroids (cortisol and adrenaline) which alter fat storage and energy balance. Chronic stress is a significant burden on the body and sets up a negative loop of reducing gut health and immunity and increasing inflammation, with a further dysregulation of hormones. High inflammation levels can negatively impact upon glands such as the thyroid. An unhappy or unhealthy gut therefore directly affects hormone levels, and gut health is important for both men and women.

During menopause poor gut health can contribute to a further loss of oestrogen and make menopause symptoms such as disrupted sleep and hot flushes worse and more frequent. Additionally, poor gut health reduces serotonin which reduces normal mood. Loss of oestrogen also reduces serotonin so poor gut health makes this loss even greater. Boosting your gut microbiome during the transition is crucial for your physical and mental health.

Self-care: Have a happy gut

- **Feed your gut microbiome.** Include probiotics that are food favourites of your gut biome and the food that probiotics like to eat, which are prebiotics. These include fermented vegetables, miso, yoghurt with live bacteria cultures and high-fibre foods.
- **Eat a rainbow.** The more differently coloured vegetables you eat the better your gut and body health – think dark leafy greens, purples, reds and orange-coloured vegetables. Ensure your daily food intake includes a diverse range of foods with high nutritional value. Think of offering your gut friends a smorgasbord of choices rather than a restricted menu.
- **Avoid damaging foods.** Some types of food, such as high-sugar foods and highly processed foods, damage your digestive system by negatively impacting your friendly gut bacteria and feeding the bad ones.

- **Reduce alcohol.** Alcohol is a natural antibacterial, which means in excess it can kill the friendly bacteria in your gut. Drinking alcohol also reduces your ability to absorb necessary vitamins and minerals essential for health and to manufacture hormones and neurotransmitters.
- **Fabulous fibre.** Fibre is an essential component in your diet. Healthy gut bacteria feast on fibre so you will be helping them help you as well as helping your body to eliminate toxins. Good sources of fibre include beans and pulses, whole grains and brown rice or a sprinkling of flaxseeds on cereal and salads. Fibre also gives you that full feeling, so you can manage portions better.
- **Move.** Physical activity and exercise help your digestive system to operate efficiently and effectively thus supporting the gut.
- **Empty your bowels.** It is necessary to eliminate your body's metabolic output. Constipation or irregular bowel movements can lead to discomfort. Although controversial, the ancient autointoxication theory posits that your health will deteriorate as you become toxic as your colon holds fermenting, decaying waste matter. Imagine not taking out household rubbish for the month. Ideally, you should eliminate your internal waste daily, and the natural response is in the morning. If you need to improve your waste management, drink more water, exercise and increase the amount of fibre you consume.

Insulin, ovaries and androgens

Insulin is the hormone that manages glucose, our primary energy source. Both the body and brain rely on glucose, which we derive from food, to function. The hormone insulin is sent from the pancreas to manage glucose in the bloodstream so there is a constant and consistent supply for every cell in the body. If there is more glucose than required it gets stored as fat, and when we eat too many high-glucose foods the insulin system gets out of kilter. The pancreas stops working effectively, either producing too little insulin and/or ineffective insulin which leads to insulin resistance.

Type II diabetes occurs when the pancreas is no longer able to function and produce enough insulin. A high-calorie diet, lack of exercise and being overweight or obese are the risk factors for type II diabetes that we can actively modify through lifestyle.

Additional risk factors for diabetes are high blood pressure (can be weight related), family history and the medical condition polycystic ovarian syndrome. Polycystic ovarian syndrome (PCOS) simply means having one or more 'cysts' on the ovaries. The term cyst is misleading as they are not in fact cysts at all but are partially formed follicles which contain our eggs. PCOS is caused by high levels of androgens – small amounts of these are usually produced in the ovaries, adrenals and fatty tissue to be converted to oestrogen, but if their levels rise to excess, due most frequently to hormone disruption, reproductive health can decline.

We do not really understand the genetic basis of PCOS, but it is likely many factors are involved such as family history, insulin resistance and lifestyle. What we do know is that it runs in families. We also know insulin resistance (diabetes) has a strong genetic factor *and* is due to lifestyle factors (weight, diet, inactivity).

High androgen levels mean lower levels of oestrogen and the loss of the wonderful health benefits it confers. This hormonal disorder affects between twelve and twenty per cent of women of reproductive age, which is significant, especially given that it reduces fertility. High levels of androgens in women can also result in increased acne, excess hair growth, high cholesterol and blood fat abnormalities, along with cardiovascular disease and endometrial carcinoma.

Another complication of high insulin levels is that oestrogen levels can *increase*, which impacts the thickness of the uterus (endometrium) and this increases the risk of endometrial cancer and breast cancer. Too much can be as dangerous as too little!

Reducing disease risk is crucial. You can't control increasing age and the menopause transition so reduce those risks you can control through lifestyle.

Self-care: Diabetes risk reduction

- **Maintain a healthy weight.** Monitor any increase in weight: it happens naturally with age and during menopause but try to remain in your healthy weight range. You may have to eat less, change what and when you eat, and increase your amount of physical exercise. Remember it is easier to lose a little weight rather than wait until you need to lose a lot.
- **Keep physically fit.** Exercise regularly: the recommendation is three hours per week so find what suits you and make it a habit. Remember walking is free and fantastic. Age and menopause change your body composition – fat storage zones change, for example – but you need to maintain muscle mass and bone density, and exercise is crucial for that. Ideally, engage in aerobic and resister exercise.
- **Eat slow-release energy foods.** Foods with a low glycaemic index, for example brown rice, brown bread, wholemeal pasta, lentils, sweet potatoes, legumes and protein of any kind, will help keep insulin levels stable. Eat less of, or avoid completely, foods that spike insulin – high-sugar foods, cakes, desserts, sweets, and white flour-based carbohydrates.
- **Reduce drinking sugar.** Drink water not soft drinks or fruit juices, which are high in sugars and are a major

contributor to obesity. Limit alcohol, as it is also high
in sugar, and high consumption of alcohol is linked to
diabetes.

- **Limit sweet treats.** Enjoy and savour 'sometimes foods',
  like dessert and special treats, but do not have them daily.
  There is no such thing as good foods and bad foods;
  rather, think of foods as sometimes foods – high in sugar,
  fat or salt – and always foods, which are healthy and
  nutritious. Stick to fresh fruit or yoghurt for dessert if
  you need to have dessert – it is an optional treat.

Alcohol and oestrogen

Women are now drinking almost as much alcohol as men. Parity
in this statistic is not liberating as alcohol affects women more
than it does men. The extent to which alcohol affects us is
dependent on a range of different factors which can be grouped
into personal (age, weight, general health, genetics), circumstances
(volume, speed and duration of alcohol consumption, food to slow
absorption, and level of dehydration), and our sex.

Alcohol research, like all medical research, traditionally used
to only include men. Today however research studies demonstrate
that women are more at risk of alcohol's toxic effects than men,
and worse, women are also more likely to develop alcohol-related
diseases sooner than men because women metabolise alcohol
differently.

There are several factors contributing to the sex-specific harm
of alcohol to women. Women tend to weigh less than men and have
more body fat. Higher body fat levels slow the metabolism of alcohol,
so it remains in the blood longer, and there is less water to dilute
alcohol. Additionally, men produce more alcohol dehydrogenase
(ADH), a group of enzymes which break down alcohol toxins
before they enter the bloodstream. As a result, women are more

likely than men to develop alcohol liver disease and more likely to die from cirrhosis of the liver as it cleans the blood.

The negative health impacts of alcohol consumption for both men and women also include: changes to blood flow, blood supply and glucose synthesis; increased cancer risk; sleep disturbance; impaired absorption of and depletion of essential vitamins and minerals; and disruption of hormone production and function and changes to fertility in both men and women. Chronic or excessive alcohol misuse by women can lead to changes in ovulation, disruption to menses, risk of miscarriage, and early menopause. Alcohol consumption leads to hypoglycaemia within six to thirty-six hours of consumption because of the spike and then drop in insulin, with between approximately forty-five and seventy per cent of people who consume excessive alcohol developing type II diabetes. Any of these effects of alcohol misuse have major implications for other medical conditions by exacerbating symptoms and inhibiting the effective treatment of them.

One area where more awareness is required is alcohol and cancer risk, especially in women. Alcohol is a known carcinogen. In women cancer is the second-highest alcohol-related health risk. A large UK study including over twenty-eight thousand women estimated that breast cancer risk begins with even low-to-moderate levels of alcohol, with every ten grams of alcohol (one standard drink) consumed per day increasing breast cancer risk by twelve per cent. Contrast this with a woman's overall lifetime risk of breast cancer, which is almost nine per cent if she drinks no alcohol. This research also suggests that women who have three alcoholic drinks *per week* have a fifteen per cent higher risk of breast cancer, and this increases exponentially with additional alcohol consumption, because alcohol increases oestrogen. Any oestrogen-dominant hormonal functions are impacted by alcohol, including PCOS, fibroids, endometriosis and hormone-receptive breast cancer. Worse, researchers have also found that alcohol diminishes the effects of an oestrogen-blocking drug widely used to treat many breast cancers.

The effect of alcohol on oestrogen levels post-menopause appears inconclusive, with some studies showing an increase, while others indicate no impact or possible *lowering*. Alcohol is a toxin with a negative impact on hormone regulation and production, including oestrogen throughout the entire lifespans of women, and when our oestrogen levels are already low in menopause it lowers them further.

Self-care: Mindful alcohol

- **Set limits.** Stick to a controlled drinking plan: determine how many days you will consume alcohol each week, and how many standard drinks you will have, and then stick to your plan. Make your alcohol consumption a conscious choice, not a habit.
- **Drink water.** Rehydrate yourself by drinking water. Drink water for thirst and before you start to consume alcohol. If you have more than one alcoholic beverage, drink water in between to help your body process the toxins and remain hydrated. Rehydrate after alcohol before you go to sleep so that your body can flush out the alcohol more easily while you are sleeping.
- **Manage the social scene.** Sometimes the hardest thing to do is not drink or not drink as much as other people as there is so much social pressure to drink alcohol! 'Hide' non-alcohol drinks in champagne flutes, wine glasses or tumblers. Carry a beer around but drink water. Be the driver and let people know you are driving. Be creative – some people need to hear a 'good' reason to respect a 'No thanks' to alcohol, and remember true friends are respectful.

- **Keep alcohol out of sight**. Having alcohol close to hand and visible increases consumption. Place bottles out of sight, pour a glass and then put the alcohol away rather than leave the bottle out or on the table. Don't keep any at home if you don't think you can ignore your home supply and only purchase alcohol for social events.
- **Eat (healthily)**. Food slows down alcohol absorption. A healthy diet also replenishes vitamins and minerals which alcohol strips out and helps maintain the gut microbiome, hormone function and general wellbeing.
- **Be active**. Alcohol can be addictive and certainly limits your capacity to engage in many activities and to be present with other people. If you find yourself drinking alone or out of boredom, perhaps develop a hobby or interest to occupy yourself and/or connect with other people.
- **Get help**. If you are concerned about your alcohol consumption, think you may have a drinking problem or any alcohol-related health issue, contact your registered medical health practitioner, drug and alcohol service, or Alcoholics Anonymous, which now runs women-only meetings.

Sleep and melatonin

We need to spend one-third of our life sleeping in order for our body and brain to go through their natural rest and restore processes to support our optimal health. Many of us experience poor sleep at times during our life, perhaps due to stress, health issues or children, and our sleep naturally changes across our lifespan, including during the menopause transition.

Our sleep–wake cycle is regulated by the body's circadian rhythm, which is governed by a tiny master clock situated in the brain's hypothalamus called the suprachiasmatic nucleus, or third eye. It directs the release of melatonin, a hormone made in the pineal gland of the brain, which helps regulate body clocks including the menstrual cycle and our sleep. Melatonin increases at night, in response to darkness, preparing the body for sleep, and declines in the early hours when cortisol gradually increases to give us the energy to get up and into the day.

During sleep we go through phases of restoration and repair. During the deepest sleep, stages three and four, most physical reparation and healing functions occur – our blood pressure has dropped, our muscles are relaxed, our heart rate drops, and our breathing rate is slow and steady. This gives our cardiovascular system time to repair and rest – without it, our risk for cardiovascular disease increases. Reduced blood use by the heart and muscles as they are relaxed during sleep means increased supply to support tissue growth and repair, including our skin – which is why so many skin products are marketed for night use. Our immune system is boosted as we produce more antibodies, and hormones are released, especially those for growth and to balance our appetite.

Although most people know they don't feel great when they are tired and recognise they need more sleep, few appreciate just how much a lack of sleep negatively impacts upon physical and mental health. Lack of sleep increases the risk of early death. It also places the body and brain under physiological stress, which impacts how well our brain functions, causing poor concentration, slower reaction speed and lack of focus. It can also cause moodiness, agitation and irritability and for some it increases risk of mental illness and psychological distress. An associated increase in cortisol reduces melatonin and sets up a negative cycle of poor sleep and increased stress, which in turn impacts hormones including serotonin, oestrogen and insulin.

Melatonin, oestrogen and serotonin are interlinked in many processes. Melatonin helps regulate oestrogen and reduces the risk of developing oestrogen-driven breast cancer by reducing cancer cell growth. Serotonin is linked to normal positive moods and declining serotonin is associated with reduced melatonin and sleep disturbance. To add to the circle, oestrogen is needed to produce serotonin. Changes in oestrogen during peri-menopause and menopause therefore impact both sleep and mood. Insomnia and sleep disorders adversely affect all aspects of health, compounding issues for women going through hormonal changes and worsening symptoms of menopause. Therefore, it is vital that women prioritise sleep and get assistance for insomnia and primary sleep disorders before peri-menopause starts.

Self-care: Sleep

- **Get the sleep you need.** Sleep is crucial for health, yet many people do not get enough. The US National Sleep Foundation recommends that adults aged twenty-six to sixty-four years have seven to nine hours per night; and those over sixty-five should aim for seven to eight hours' sleep each night. It takes time to fall asleep – allow fifteen to thirty minutes. Don't force sleep, or stress if you can't get to sleep easily and within that time. Try something relaxing like reading or meditation for a while and start again.
- **Confine day sleeps.** A siesta is a great concept, but an afternoon nap can interfere with your ability to sleep at night. If you do like a power nap make sure you keep it short – up to thirty minutes – and make sure it is around midday to work with your body's natural rhythm, not late in the afternoon.
- **Stick to a routine.** Have a regular sleep and wake time as this gives your body and brain the signals for sleep. It takes two hours for melatonin levels to build up for sleep

(and for cortisol to increase for waking), so develop a routine. Not having a regular sleep and wake program gets the entire rhythm out of kilter. Also establish a pre-sleep routine as this cues the brain to prepare for sleep.

- **Limit body tasks.** Our body needs to restore and then rest and recharge when we sleep. Eating a large meal before bed reduces sleep as your body needs to digest rather than rest. Similarly, if you need to get up to toilet at night consider limiting how much you drink in the few hours before sleep time so you do not disrupt your sleep cycles with toilet breaks.
- **The right light.** Our brain responds to light. The blue light of day increases cortisol output for energy, while red or orange light linked to night stimulates melatonin for sleep. Turn screens and devices to night mode and turn down bedroom lights or use nightlights. In the morning open blinds/curtains/window coverings and look at the natural light.
- **Exercise.** Being physically active and exercising during the day helps with sleep, as you become physically tired and any excess stress in the system is depleted. Exercise also reduces fatigue during the day by giving you more energy, and it helps reduce the likelihood of weight gain, which is associated with lack of sleep.
- **Get cool and comfortable.** To sleep, our body temperature needs to drop. You can assist by showering, wearing cool clothes, and keeping bedrooms cool and/or having windows open for air flow. Make sure the room is dark and stays dark. Block out ambient light and remove devices that flash. Get the best pillow and mattress you can to suit your body.
- **Avoid stimulants.** Caffeine, smoking and alcohol all reduce our capacity to fall asleep and stay asleep.

Excessive garlic and chilli in your meal may also keep you awake as they increase body temperature. Stimulants increase night sweats and hot flushes. Dairy products before bedtime can assist sleep – but in moderation.

Summary: Enhancing hormone health

Hormones are complicated messengers essential for health. Our lifestyles affect the production and regulation of hormones, so rather than just relying on medication or supplements, target your lifestyle. Take out the negative habits and add in positive beneficial ones. Now is the perfect time to launch your optimal health habits to manage menopause symptoms and boost general health to ensure you thrive.

- **Improve your gut health.** Care for your gut health by consuming healthy nutritious foods, fibre, prebiotics and probiotics to improve your production and regulation of key hormones such as serotonin, insulin, ghrelin and leptin. Manage stress and limit sugar, alcohol and recreational drugs as they decrease gut health.
- **Keep a healthy weight.** As we age it is important to stay at our ideal weight, or get to a healthy weight, for multiple health benefits. Weight loss becomes harder with age and menopause, and some natural weight gain (~three kilograms) is normal in menopause, so be sure your weight is healthy beforehand. Excess fat, however, increases oestrogen production and disrupts the balance between oestrogen and progesterone. The excess of oestrogen worsens PMS and increases cancer risk.
- **Eat healthy fats and oils.** Our bodies require various types of fats to produce hormones, reduce inflammation, boost metabolism and promote weight loss. Healthy oils

are unsaturated and include avocados, and nut and olive oils.

- **Increase omega 3.** Good sources of omega 3 are wild fish, walnuts, flaxseeds, grass-fed animal products and eggs. It is also important to decrease omega 6 fats such as those in red meat and in corn, cotton seed, soybean, peanut and canola oils.

- **Capture some rays.** Vitamin D is essential for optimal health and does a lot more than increase the absorption of calcium. Vitamin D acts more like a hormone and supports many bodily processes, such as increasing the absorption of nutrients and reducing disease risks including some cancers and osteoporosis. The best source is the sun so get outside and expose your arms and/or legs to the sun for ten to twenty minutes mid-morning or mid-afternoon.

- **Exercise.** As mentioned before, exercise has multiple health benefits. Being fit and strong will boost metabolism, bones, heart health and brain function. It is also instrumental in balancing hormones such as insulin and cortisol, and promoting sleep, and releases beneficial endorphins, dopamine, growth hormones and testosterone, and increases immunity.

- **Reduce stress.** Chronic levels of stress are a health hazard. All the strategies listed here assist your body to better manage stress, but you may need to also address the cause. Take time out for yourself. Develop problem-solving strategies, share your problems and recruit help, change your thinking, focus on priorities, learn relaxation, and seek professional help if necessary.

- **Improve your sleep.** A lack of sleep impacts our entire bodies and brains. It can also change the blood serum levels of multiple hormones and increases our susceptibility to stress. Stick to the schedule I talked about earlier (see pages 43–7), and consider taking melatonin.

- **Avoid stimulants.** Stimulants such as alcohol, caffeine and nicotine are all problematic for hormone function, with smokers estimated to reach menopause almost two years earlier than non-smokers. Similarly, avoid non-prescription and recreational drugs.

- **Review oral contraception.** The types of oral contraceptives that significantly increase oestrogen levels have been linked to increased risk of breast cancer, depression, weight gain and other health problems. There are other ways not to get pregnant that don't affect your natural hormone balance. Where hormone treatments are necessary find the one that works best for your needs – there are plenty of options available – support your hormone health with lifestyle strategies and monitor hormone use over your lifespan.

- **Eliminate toxins.** Drinking water, eating fibre and exercising helps your body eliminate toxins and have regular bowel motions. You can also help by reducing your exposure to harmful toxins in products and the environment. Beauty care products are full of harmful substances including DEA (diethanolamine), parabens, sodium lauryl sulphate and propylene glycol. Reconsider your beauty regime. Think about reducing your exposure plastics. Consider using glassware and not plastic for food and drink storage or heating. Perhaps even review clothes and furniture and other products that you use in your home. Keep outdoor shoes outdoors, as we walk in heavy metals and other toxins without knowing it.

- **Love your liver.** Your liver is fundamental to your health as it filters the blood coming from your gut before it goes to the rest of your body, clearing toxins. It removes cholesterol, used hormones, drugs, alcohol, bilirubin; it activates enzymes; it metabolises fats, proteins and carbohydrates; it stores vitamins and minerals; and it syntheses plasma proteins. Eat lots of cruciferous vegetables, such as broccoli, Brussels sprouts, cabbage and cauliflower, to support these functions.

- **Balance your body.** Make sure that your essential vitamin and mineral levels are at the right balance so your brain and body can produce all the hormones and neurotransmitters you need. Vitamin D, Vitamin B12 and iron, for example, ensure normal energy levels, brain function and mood. The best way to get the balance is to make sure every meal is highly nutritious, and to eat diverse foods and vegetables, and only take supplements if you have a deficiency.

- **Keep health checks up to date.** Age, menopausal changes and a combination of both impact other health conditions so it is vital to keep health checks and screens up to date. Consider monitoring breast, bone, cervix, bowel and eye health as well as cholesterol, insulin, blood pressure and weight.

- **Be proactive.** If you have concerns about the health of your hormones see your nominated treating health practitioners. You can have a comprehensive blood test to check hormones such as Vitamin D, or saliva hormone profiling to measure cortisol, for example, or for a big picture view try hormone symptom profiling. Be wary of any health practitioners who 'diagnose' a health issue and then directly profit from the supplement treatment they recommend. Receive the diagnosis and then purchase products somewhere else.

Glossary of key hormones and health hints to support them

Adrenal glands: are two endocrine glands which sit one above each kidney and produce several hormones, including adrenaline and the steroid cortisol. They are sometimes called the adrenal cortex because of the direct communication they have with the brain via the HPA axis (hypothalamus–pituitary–adrenal group). The adrenal glands produce androgens and after menopause some of these are converted to oestrogen. It is important to support adrenal function by keeping stress levels low, so that the adrenal glands produce important hormones and not just cortisol. Be mindful not to engage in constant or excessive aerobic exercise as this can become a burden, and make sure you allow complete recovery time, and make sure you consume vitamin C.

Adrenaline (epinephrine): an amino acid hormone secreted by the adrenal glands that increases rates of blood pressure to boost circulation, breathing and carbohydrate metabolism, and which prepares muscles for exertion. Adrenaline is associated with the stress response. The concept of low adrenal reserve, or adrenal insufficiency, remains inconclusive, and is said to occur when the adrenals no longer produce enough adrenalin to meet bodily demand. This may arise because of prolonged stress (due to emotional, medical/viral and/or physical demands). 'Adrenal support' involves reduction of stress and comprises adequate rest, gentle exercise, high nutrition, and if necessary supplementation with physician guidance.

Allopregnanolone: a progesterone derivative that has similar sedative effects to those achieved by taking benzodiazepines. It is termed an endogenous inhibitory neuro-steroid – meaning it is self-made and has a calming effect on the brain.

Androgens: a chemical class of different steroid hormones in men and women including testosterone and DHEA (dehydro-epiandrosterone), which stimulate growth, muscles, bones, etc.

The primary group of androgens are the adrenal androgens. Androstenedione is produced in the adrenal glands, testes and ovaries and adipose tissue and is converted to other androgens such as oestrogen. High stress compromises the ability to make androgens as too much adrenaline is produced instead. Managing stress is vital to keep the right balance of androgens. In women androgens are also produced in the ovaries and fat cells.

Antidiuretic hormone (ADH): regulates water balance in the body, conserving body water by increasing the amount of reabsorption thus reducing the amount lost in urine. It is also involved in blood pressure regulation as it constricts blood flow (increasing blood pressure) and hence it is also called vasopressin.

Cortisol: a steroid hormone that energises you to get you up in the morning. Like adrenaline it regulates the stress response and is also produced by the adrenal glands. Cortisol influences stress glucose metabolism and immune function. However, excessive cortisol becomes a burden on the body and brain as it has a catabolic (breaking down) action on body tissue, leading to low immunity, allergies, stress-related illness and brain changes. Stress management is crucial to turn down cortisol.

DHEA (dehydroepiandrosterone): this hormone is a pre-androgen in both men and women and produced primarily by the adrenal glands. It converts to androgens and oestrogens in women and testosterone in men. Its synthesis influences energy, stamina, mental outlook and immune function, and for these reasons it is also known as the anti-aging hormone. Evidence also suggests it helps alleviate depression and regulates the effects of excess cortisol.

Dopamine: a neurotransmitter produced in several areas of the brain; it only works within the brain. Dopamine is crucial to reward and pleasure, and is therefore involved in motivating behaviour, giving reward and supporting learning. It also helps regulate movement and emotional responses. Dopamine makes us feel great after sex, being with friends, eating chocolate, dancing or engaging in other enjoyable healthy activities. Dopamine is also elevated after taking psychoactive substances, such as alcohol and recreational drugs. Excessive artificial peaks of dopamine can lead to addiction.

Endorphins: the word is an abbreviation of endogenous morphine, which essentially means 'naturally produced painkiller'. They are a group of peptide neurohormones that work within the brain to block pain reception thereby having an analgesic effect. They also have an opiate effect that produces positive feelings, even euphoria, and energisation. Exercise is a great natural way to boost endorphins.

Follicle stimulating hormone (FSH): is released by the pituitary gland and triggers ovulation in women and the production of sperm in men. It goes up and down to give us our menstrual cycle. Elevated levels may mark the onset of menopause as there are few eggs left in the ovaries.

Ghrelin: the 'hunger hormone', a peptide hormone mainly made in the stomach to stimulate appetite – when the stomach is empty it is secreted and tells the brain you are hungry and then the brain motivates you to get food. Feeling a little hungry before eating is a healthy normal response – don't panic. If you are not hungry ask why you are eating. Ghrelin also regulates distribution of energy use and the secretion of the growth hormone from the pituitary gland.

Growth hormone: made in the pituitary gland, it stimulates growth and cell reproduction which helps maintain our entire body. For this reason, it is also termed the elixir of youth. The amount of growth hormones you have circulating depends a lot on how much quality sleep you have, so maintain a good sleep regimen.

Hyperthyroidism: is when the thyroid gland is overactive. *See also* Thyroid.

Hypothalamus: among its roles the hypothalamus acts as the relay station between the brain and central nervous system and the hormone endocrine system. The hypothalamus allows the brain and body to 'talk' to each other. It governs physiological processes – sleep, temperature, sex drive, hunger and thirst, for example. It is also part of the hypothalamus–pituitary–adrenal axis (HPA) feedback system involved in the stress response. Maintain optimal health to help this and other key players of the endocrine system.

Hypothyroidism: is low thyroid function, often associated with hormonal imbalance (particularly oestrogen dominance) and linked with cold body temperature (feeling cold all the time), weight gain, an inability to lose weight, thinning hair, low libido and depression. Women are at greatest risk, developing thyroid problems seven times more often than men, particularly during the years prior to menopause. *See also* Thyroid.

Insulin: is made and regulated by the pancreas under the direction of the pituitary gland to manage blood glucose levels and glycogenesis, lipids and the synthesis of fatty acids. Glucagon also assists to regulate blood sugar levels. Stress limits the impact of insulin while stress hormones rise.

Insulin resistance: a term used to describe the failure of the tissues to respond (resistance) to insulin and absorb glucose for energy production; this is associated with hormonal imbalance (particularly high triglycerides, polycystic ovaries and excess androgens). Insulin resistance leads to increased risk of cardiovascular disease, diabetes and cancer. Maintain a healthy weight and eat a highly nutritious balanced diet with few added sugary or highly processed foods.

Leptin: is secreted by body fat (adipose tissue), and acts to decrease appetite and increase metabolism. It has a major role in fat storage, appetite and energy regulation and inhibits hunger when we have enough stored energy. Always listen to your body rather than overriding what it is telling you. If you feel full, stop eating. Eat meals slowly and savour your food – that way you can enjoy your food more and give your body time to say, 'Enough'. Exercise and having high muscle mass also help to boost metabolism. Sleep well, as insufficient and poor-quality sleep affects insulin and leptin and increases fat storage and the risk for metabolic disorders.

Luteinising hormone (LH): is released by the pituitary gland and in women signals ovulation and to make progesterone. In men, it signals the testes to produce testosterone. Levels may rise during menopause.

Melatonin: the sleep hormone is produced in the pineal gland in the brain and is the hormone that helps you sleep by regulating the circadian rhythm (the body's 24-hour clock). As the sun goes down, your cortisol levels will naturally decrease (unless you are stressed), triggering your body to produce more melatonin. Shift workers, international travellers and others with disturbed sleep may be given supplements with physician guidance. Having a regular sleep time and reducing light help set the routine production of melatonin for a natural sleep cycle. Increasing melatonin can increases serotonin.

Oestrogens (estrogens): a family of three hormones (oestradiol, oestrone and oestriol) released by the ovaries. Optimal health – including being a healthy weight – is necessary for oestrogen.

Oestrogen dominance: an excess of oestrogen in the absence of adequate levels of progesterone in women (or testosterone in men). It can result from oestrogen replacement therapy, menopause, hysterectomy, birth control pills and/or a decline in ovarian progesterone production. In men, it can be the result of reduced testosterone production by the testes. In either gender, it can result from exposure to pollutants and toxins (xenoestrogens). The constellation of symptoms ranges from breast tenderness and bloating to mood swings and depression. Excess oestrogens are a risk factor for the development of breast and prostate cancers.

Oxytocin: is known as the love hormone. It is a peptide hormone and a neuropeptide, meaning it communicates between brain cells and within the body and is produced in the hypothalamus. Originally, it was thought to be present only during childbirth and involved in milk flow, but it is now known to play other roles in sexual reproduction and relationships including orgasm, bonding, trust and secure attachment, social behaviour and facial expression recognition. Oxytocin is now given as a nasal spray for children with autism to help them interpret facial expressions and develop social skills. Oxytocin makes us feel secure, loved and lovable. A ten-second hug along with other forms of physical contact will trigger the release of oxytocin. Consider arranging a massage if you are isolated and have no hugs available, as this kind of human contact also promotes oxytocin production.

Pancreas: sits above the stomach and assists digestion by producing enzymes and hormones. It is also responsible for the production of insulin and glucagon to regulate blood glucose levels. When the pancreas is unable to produce enough and/or sufficient quality insulin, type II diabetes mellitus develops. A healthy diet with limited added sugar keeps it working well.

Pineal gland: also known as the pineal body, it sits in the middle of the brain like the third eye and is the major site of melatonin production for sleep as part of the body's daily cycle or circadian rhythm.

Pituitary gland: it's only pea-sized but this gland in the brain is a major endocrine player; it produces several types of hormones that trigger and regulate other endocrine glands and the steroid hormones.

Progesterone: is a female steroid hormone released by the ovaries and adrenal glands (and placenta during pregnancy); it is essential for conception and the maintenance of pregnancy. It builds the endometrium, makes cervical mucus permeable to sperm, inhibits the immune response against the embryo and inhibits labour. It is also involved in other essential body functions and mood.

Progestin: synthetic hormones structurally similar to progesterone (for example, Provera) but not naturally occurring in the body; they suppress normal ovarian production of progesterone and have been shown in studies to have negative side effects.

Prolactin: stimulates milk production in the mammary glands after childbirth. It also affects sex hormone levels and sexual gratification after intercourse.

Serotonin: is a neurotransmitter and hormone vital for normal mood along with social behaviour and cyclic energy. It is made in the brain and the gastrointestinal tract through a biochemical conversion process. As serotonin is important for normal mood, many antidepressants increase the amount of serotonin in the brain. Levels of serotonin increase with exposure to natural light, exercise, a healthy diet and positive thinking – which can be difficult at first, so start with the lifestyle changes and the mindstyle changes will be easier. Poor gut health reduces serotonin so eat a healthy diet and decrease sugar and stress. Serotonin is a precursor to melatonin.

Testosterone: is considered the male sex hormone but women have testosterone too, released by the ovaries and adrenal glands. It is a steroid hormone and governs libido, vitality and confidence in both men and women. It also plays a role in bone health, muscle mass and skin elasticity, as well as the cardiovascular system. Low testosterone levels lead to loss of libido, loss of muscle mass, an increase in fatty tissue, and a general loss of drive and enthusiasm.

Thyroid: a major gland of the endocrine system that produces hormones, of which the main ones are thyroxine and triiodothyronine, to regulate your metabolism and energy production. Indications that your thyroid is out of whack and under-functioning are cold hands and feet, excess weight, hair loss, tiredness and low mood especially in the latter part of the day. An overactive thyroid is less common. Eat protein-rich foods with zinc, iodine and selenium.

Thyroid-stimulating hormone (TSH): stimulates the thyroid gland to produce thyroid hormones, which regulate the body's metabolism, energy balance, growth, and nervous system activity, and is regulated by the hypothalamus and anterior pituitary gland.

Xenoestrogens: are chemical compounds that imitate oestrogen. These may be either natural or synthetic and are increasingly used in plastics, herbicides, pesticides, dry-cleaning chemicals and other chemicals, birth control pills, cosmetics and food products. They have been linked to numerous reproductive disorders and cancers so be aware and reduce your exposure where you can. Use natural beauty products, avoid nail polish, air out dry-cleaned items before use, and use glassware not plastic to store food. Help the liver clear xenoestrogens by consuming antioxidant-rich foods, drinking water and resisting alcohol and smoking.

PART 3

THE
CHANGE

Menopause is a healthy and normal part of women's lives, shifting their bodies from cycling hormones for fertility to hormone stability for health maintenance. Unless it is medical or surgical menopause, it takes time, with most women experiencing changes in their bodies years before their periods finally cease.

Case study: A short story

I had a period and then it just stopped for three months.
Then one day I had a very heavy period for one day and then never again.
I had no menopause symptoms.

The pause in menses is not officially diagnosed menopause until a woman has had no period for twelve months and occurs when women are around age fifty-one. Before age forty-five the loss of menses is often called early menopause, and before age forty is called premature menopause, although the term primary oestrogen insufficiency is also used. For those nearing age sixty the term late menopause is given. The time before menopause when hormones are fluctuating wildly is termed peri-menopause and usually starts in the mid-forties. The time after menopause is called post-menopause but is the same as menopause.

Menopause can last from months to years with some women experiencing ongoing symptoms for decades, like one seventy-odd-year-old I know. Eventually for most women, however, their bodies adjust to a new level of hormonal stability. Women are now increasingly taking ownership of the term post-menopause to describe the time when they have no more symptoms of menopause and are focusing on the positive liberating aspects of hormone stability.

Menopause as a reproductive stage, therefore, has three phases: peri-menopause, menopause and post-menopause. A common term, and the one favoured here, is the collective term menopause transition. This more accurately captures the nature of the change as a process and the stages before, during and after our periods finally stop. With care and a focus on your health the menopause transition can become a time of improved wellbeing and personal growth, a midlife stage from which to spring into the next twenty to thirty years of post-menopause life.

In western societies menopause has often been portrayed negatively and as a result some women may feel trepidation and dread regarding menopause and increasing age, or perhaps have unrealistic or negative expectations. Attitudes towards menopause have a significant impact on how women experience the transition and how they cope and manage. Let's change the story of menopause for women – after all, menopause is a natural process of being healthy and ought to be celebrated. Our bodies are simply changing from being ruled by cyclical sex hormones for reproduction to purely hormonal health maintenance. This new hormone stability provides us with the opportunity for growth as we can channel our energy into the next stage of our lives and make some time for ourselves. Menopause liberates us from sexual reproduction and enables us to carry on with our dreams into a new future.

Science bite: Evolution of menopause

Humans are unique in that the female of the species ceases to be fertile while still healthy. In animals fertility continues into older age until ill health takes over and death quickly follows. Many have wondered why humans are different. The popular evolutionary explanation is that as complex highly sociable beings, child-rearing requires multiple generations to secure survival and success. Specifically, help from grandmothers. Men do not experience total loss of fertility until they die, although increasing age in men increases the risks of birth and development issues in offspring. Menopause stops women from having more children of their own, so they are free to help their children have children. Studies of original cultures confirm that in those families and societies where grandmothers are involved in raising children the survival rates of children significantly improve. Whole communities benefit too with increased labour and food gathering capacity. By becoming incapable of having children, older women are unencumbered and able to assist in the care of their grandchildren or children generally, and/or contribute to their communities.

The other possible but less romantic explanation for menopause is we live too long.

Peri-menopause

Peri-menopause often creeps up on us, as we can be unaware of hormonal changes until the cycling levels of oestrogen and progesterone become desynchronised and we experience symptoms. Often the first symptom of the transition women notice is a change to their menstrual cycle or quality of their periods which may become shorter, longer, heavier, lighter, closer together, further apart, and generally irregular.

The general lowering of oestrogen and progesterone, and the ratios between them, affects other systems. Night sweats, hot flushes and poor sleep may start, as these symptoms don't wait for menopause proper to begin. However, the symptoms and signs of peri-menopause are not necessarily consistent, making it hard to recognise what is happening. Periods can suddenly cease – as with the woman in 'A short story' – gradually fade out, become erratic and unpredictable, flood, dribble, or change pattern continuously.

Much like menopause, women often don't talk about periods. This can make it hard to know if you are experiencing 'normal' periods or peri-menopausal changes or symptoms of something more serious. It is very easy to think that your natural cycle is normal or that the nature of your periods is normal. It is very common for women to tolerate heavy periods and do nothing. Menorrhagia is the medical term for heavy bleeding and is indicated if you need to change your sanitary items every hour or two for two or more hours. In my own health journey, I had no idea I was in that class and my doctor was horrified that I had coped with it for as long as I had. If you are experiencing changes such as heavy bleeding, spotting, periods longer than seven days, cramps and abdominal pain, I implore you to please speak up and seek help. Iron deficiency is a risk but there may also be other medical conditions, such as fibroids, endometriosis and possibly uterine cancer, which need to be treated.

Science bite: Follicle loss leads to menopause

Menopause is a normal physiological event brought about by the loss of ovarian follicular function – essentially it means no more eggs. Through the process of continuous depletion called atresia, the human ovary steadily loses follicles. As fewer remain there is less stimulation of the gran cells and lower and lower levels of oestrogen being secreted.

In an attempt to compensate the anterior pituitary gland responds by releasing more FSH to stimulate more follicles to mature and increase the production of oestrogen. This ultimately exhausts the system as the follicles become insensitive and do not mature. However, there can be transient increases and surges in oestrogen. As the follicles do not mature there is less progesterone. This causes the huge fluctuations of oestrogen and progesterone during peri-menopause and are much greater than the cyclical changes that occur during normal phases of the menstrual cycle. Once there are no more follicles menstruation ceases completely and menopause is determined after twelve months.

Women's fertility starts to slowly decline from our mid-twenties and drops quite steeply after our mid-thirties. Noticeable or reported changes in the menstrual cycle naturally begin when women are in their forties, with forty-six being the average age for onset of peri-menopause in Australian women. Despite these statistics, I know of women in their late forties whose treating doctors have dismissed their suggestion that they were in peri-menopause and some even suggested that peri-menopause did not exist. The fact that puberty takes many years would suggest that its opposite, the ending of periods, would also take time and need to start before menopause at age fifty-one. On average, peri-menopause appears to take four years, although there is huge variation from a few months to ten years.

Most women can easily recognise changes within themselves as they know their body, its signs and patterns best. But for health professionals recognising peri-menopause is not an easy task as they cannot see what is going on. Doctors and other health professionals are most likely to make a 'diagnosis' based upon the symptoms that women report. It is possible to have a blood test that measures levels of oestrogen and/or FSH to check how much of these hormones are still being produced. However, as your hormone levels are fluctuating daily, possibly wildly with peri-menopause, a blood test on a single day will only give you a record for that day and not accurately record hormone levels in a reliable or meaningful way. Blood tests may be effective if multiple tests are taken at different times over several days, which is not very feasible.

The problem, though, is that when a single blood test comes back normal it is too easy to say there are no changes and the symptom reports of women may not be taken seriously. I know a woman who at age forty-nine went to a doctor for blood tests to confirm that she was in peri-menopause. One blood test was taken, and the doctor determined that she could not be peri-menopausal. She changed doctors. She knew herself. She had enjoyed very regular monthly periods without oral contraception for decades and knew that having only nine periods in one year was a sure sign of something. Women don't need someone else to tell them their periods are changing – they know – but a good differential diagnosis is necessary to make sure that this is part of the natural transition process and not something more complicated. It is important to state that although irregular periods are normal and common during peri-menopause, there are other medical conditions that can cause you to miss a few periods, such as hormone problems, pregnancy, issues with contraception, blood clotting and, although uncommon, cancer.

If you are experiencing changes and think you may have embarked on the menopause transition, or are having issues, a good place to start is to know yourself. Keep track of all the changes you are noticing – what they are and when they occur. Using a diary will help keep track of frequency and duration and make it easier to develop a big-picture view. Rate how much each change or issue is a problem – it is possible that symptoms do not bother you! Write down what you think might be triggering them – diet, time, stress, etc and any solutions that you have tried. If you try something to alleviate the issue stick to it for at least a few weeks as it can take time for treatment or lifestyle changes to make a difference.

Additionally, the chaos of fluctuating levels of oestrogen and progesterone has implications for fertility. You may not always have a period, but you may have still ovulated. Or you may have a period and you might not always ovulate, as the ovaries might not release a matured egg and instead resorb it back into the body. The lack of clear messages from your body regarding its fertility has serious implications for birth control and fertility. Check contraception as necessary and review fertility if that is your concern.

Peri-menopause, and menopause, are entirely unpredictable. The experience of our mothers is no guide either. The start and nature of our periods throughout our lives also has no bearing on their fluctuation and cessation. Many factors, including lifestyle ones, influence the onset of peri-menopause and the transition experience, as well as the impact upon other systems such as vascular function, bone health and oestrogen-sensitive brain circuits.

Case study: Masked menopause

I discovered I was peri-menopausal when I had my Mirena IUD taken out at age thirty-seven so my husband and I could try for a third child. With two immediately conceived pregnancies behind me, I'd assumed the third would be simple.

But a few days later I started having irregular cycles – three days, then forty days, then sixteen days – ending with heavy bleeding.

I went to a fertility specialist with my blood and ultrasound tests, and she told me I had the reproductive system of a woman in her late fifties. The hormones from the Mirena had masked my ebbing cycles, and she estimated I had less than five per cent chance of having another child. The reason she gave me even five per cent was because I'd had two successful pregnancies. IVF was pointless since I had few follicles to recruit.

I found myself staring with blistering envy at pregnant women on the train, in the playground, at the gym. I was confused and guilty about the oceanic sadness that filled me. We already had two healthy boys. Why was I so greedy?

At the same time as I saw these blooming, sanguine women everywhere, my own body was faltering. 'Menopause' was such an ugly, old, wrinkled word. Was I becoming ugly, old and wrinkled too? I would stare into the mirror with horror, noting the pillowing softness around my middle where I'd never had softness before. My breasts looked empty and my nipples seemed shrivelled. I experienced vaginal dryness. I had days and nights of intense hot flushes which drove me to despair. I would wake with a sick jolt of terror as if someone had stuck a gun to my temple in my sleep, and the familiar burning sensation would crawl across my skin. Menopause was making me an old woman in my thirties.

The fertility specialist had explained I might have one or two normal ovulations in the next year or two but couldn't say what quality those last eggs would be. At thirty-seven they might be viable.

I grew obsessive about those last eggs. I hunched over my laptop, suffering hot flushes as I scoured fertility sites like a crazy woman. I took my basal body temperature every morning to chart if I was ovulating at all. I tried to predict my rare ovulations, but it was futile when they were so capricious. In the end I decided the best way to get pregnant was to have sex at least every other day so if a precious, viable egg arrived, my husband's sperm would be waiting.

After a few months of this, my husband and I found ourselves wishing we could spend our evenings watching a gentle nature documentary over a cup of tea.

Ten months later, I was becoming accustomed to the idea I'd be a mother of two. I was getting comfortable with the symptoms of peri-menopause. We were lucky, and our family was solid. We'd toss this stressful regime of sex after my next non-cycle.

Then after eleven months, as I was buttering toast one morning, I felt a familiar queasy gurgle. My fingers were shaking as I held the test under the brightest lamp in the house and saw the faint pink line. That test heralded the beginning of my daughter's life. She's now three.

I'm forty-three and almost through menopause now. I still have hot flushes and other symptoms, but the word 'menopause' doesn't make me shudder any more. We got our third child by some wondrous cosmic fluke, and the rest I'll live with, or manage with HRT.

Menopause

Count twelve months of no period and you can claim you are in menopause, unless you have had a hysterectomy and there is no such obvious indicator. With menopause, the fluctuations of oestrogen and progesterone have ceased and your body is adjusting to lower levels of less potent oestrogen. Yes, we still have oestrogen, as it is necessary to maintain our health, but we now rely on a different form made in different places in our bodies, and in much lower quantities than before. Our bodies now rely on oestrogen in the same way as men's bodies have always done.

The changes and symptoms women experience during the transition are due to the loss of the supercharged source of oestrogen (and progesterone and testosterone) and adaptation to a new limited and weaker form. And we do adapt, with the majority of women managing very well. It just takes time. Sometimes there may be so many other things going on in life that the absence of periods is not even noticed. Or those things going on may explain the loss of regular periods – late unexpected pregnancy, illness, severe stress or rapid weight loss. Other times, life events of much greater significance unfold and menopause by comparison is not even worth mentioning. The changes are the same, but the symptoms and experience of the transition vary considerably.

Case study: Menopause mayhem

I met my partner when I was thirty-seven and he forty. Neither of us had children but three years later that all changed. I had two miscarriages then found out I was pregnant. We had a beautiful son, but life quickly proved challenging for him, and in turn for us. He didn't sleep during the day at all and barely slept at night. We finally discovered he had intolerance to many foods. He was in fact constantly in pain and screaming. While this chaos was happening in my life my father was told there was nothing more that could be done to treat the cancer that was taking

70

over his body. I was sleep deprived ... feeling desperate ... needing help with my child ... feeling grief for my dad and helplessness for mum. Life felt surreal and my emotions were all over the place.

I was only able to breastfeed for the first six weeks, so my menstrual cycle started up again not long after feeding stopped. For the next sixteen months my cycle remained irregular. I had night sweats and foggy brain and moods, which my doctor all put down to having a newborn and stress.

I felt I was not in control of my life ... but there seemed to be no obvious explanations for my feeling so scrambled. I saw my GP regularly (usually with my screaming child due to his latest bout of diarrhoea and eczema) and I would often end up a bucket of tears. I mentioned my symptoms. She felt St John's wort was needed for my state of mind – or lack of it! She was sure it was all sleep deprivation, stress and grief. I took the pills every day for three months and saw my doctor to talk about me. I had isolated myself from friends and family as I was ashamed I wasn't able to cope.

At home I felt completely alone – my partner didn't understand. He ran his own business and is a very self-contained person – this really wasn't how he had imagined family life. This period of my life – which felt like I was existing and not living – took another turn when at forty-two I found out I was expecting another child. I was elated but also concerned. My son's health issues were still affecting his life so negatively and dictating mine too as I was spending every waking moment with an assortment of health professionals. Feelings of joy were quickly overridden by those concerns. The main thing I noticed about this pregnancy was how well I felt – the night sweats, foggy brain and mood swings seemed to disappear.

I had my daughter four months after my forty-third birthday and she was a breeze. No complicated health or developmental issues. Having a completely different child made me realise it wasn't my crappy parenting that was to blame for my son's litany of health issues – as there were many times that I had blamed myself as the cause of his problems. About four months after having my daughter I started experiencing night sweats and flushing again. My vagina was as dry as the Sahara Desert and my sex drive was in hiding. I had recently had a baby, so all these symptoms were understandable.

It was not until I started asking doctors 'Could I be going through menopause?' and after being told 'You don't need to worry, you've just had a baby,' that I was finally sent for an ultrasound of my ovaries. Lying there having the procedure I was told I had the ovaries of a seventy-year-old! Blood tests followed, and all was confirmed. I obviously started menopause after having my son but did not notice, and my daughter was probably my last egg!

Was menopause brought on relatively early due to stress? No one knows. By the time I had answers I had been through three years of menopause symptoms unaware that they were contributing to the way I was mentally and physically feeling. In a way it was a relief. The rest of my menopause journey was relatively uneventful, and I managed the remaining few years that I suffered flushes and sweats, and ever-changing energy levels, with over-the-counter menopause treatments and diet.

Unfortunately, there were few to share my experiences with. None of my girlfriends were at that stage in their lives; my sister is younger and my darling mother, quite Victorian in her attitude to female health, wouldn't say. In a funny way I found the information of my menopause status empowering – I had unknowingly got through such a tumultuous period of my life and I had managed ... at times not very well, but I got through and I did realise I needed to be kinder to myself.

When our ovaries stop producing oestradiol for sexual reproduction they continue to make a form of oestrogen known as oestrone, but not all that we require. We produce approximately half our oestrone in the adrenal glands and in adipose tissue (including breast tissue), like men and children do. This form of oestrogen has very specific targeted functions and its production is related to where it is used, such as in the aortic smooth muscle cells to maintain cardiovascular function and in numerous sites in the brain for brain function. If we do not produce enough oestrone during menopause then the symptoms of menopause will be worse.

This change in oestrogen type, potency, volume and production sites leads to a disruption in an entire chain of biochemical activities, and affects the production and regulation of other hormones, including those mood-regulating ones like serotonin, endorphins and oxytocin. If you skipped Part 2 on hormone health I suggest you go back and familiarise yourself with hormone basics because overall hormone health is essential to have sufficient oestrone.

The hormone changes impact cells, organs and systems such as our level of hydration, smooth muscles, the vascular system and bone density. There are dozens of symptoms linked to these changes, including headaches, hot flushes, fatigue, osteoporosis, interrupted sleep, vaginal dryness, loss of libido, mental confusion, lowered concentration and mood swings.

Science bite: Post-menopause oestrogen production

Ovaries share the production of oestrone (E_1) with the adrenal glands and adipose tissue (fatty tissues) by converting androgens produced by the adrenal glands into oestrogen using the hormone aromatase, found in fatty tissue.

Oestrogen use now becomes site specific. In the fatty adipose tissue of the breasts, oestrogen acts on mesenchymal stem cells, which means that they can become other cell types for specific purposes such as: osteoblasts (bone cells), chondrocytes (cartilage cells) and myocytes (muscle cells). Where oestrogen is produced in bone, the osteoblasts and chondrocytes support bone mineralisation and, therefore, reduce osteoporosis. In the smooth muscle cells of the aorta and in the vascular endothelium, oestrogen acts to support the vascular system. Because the oestrogen is now primarily site specific there is very limited oestrogen circulating in the body and, therefore, it has very limited influence on the amount in any one site. As a result, it is possible to have too much oestrogen at one site but not have enough elsewhere. For example, you can have too much in the breast and develop breast cancer, but have very low levels of oestrogen to support bone health.

To try to make sense of all the symptoms of change, and other health issues that can arise, I have divided the changes into the broad categories of: body, brain and mind, and relationships. However, this categorisation is purely arbitrary, and there is considerable crossover between them as they are all inextricably linked. The reality for each of us is that our experience of the menopause transition is uniquely personal and determined by multiple factors. Each of us, and those who love us, needs to navigate this phase the best way possible and having a positive and accepting attitude improves the journey.

Science bite: Decline in the big three

Oestrogen Reduction in oestrogen leads to disruption to fluid balance, blood coagulation and cholesterol, bone density and smooth muscle, with symptoms of headaches, fatigue, hot flushes, joint pain and memory lapses. Lower levels of oestrogen are also linked to increases in cortisol, which impacts mood and mental health.

Progesterone As oestrogen declines so does progesterone. Its loss is associated with headaches, along with muscle weakness, irregular heartbeat, vaginal infections, mood swings and anxiety. Research into the impact on the brain is only just beginning.

Testosterone The 'male' hormone drops with increasing age and decreasing fertility. By the time women are in natural menopause, levels have dropped by twenty per cent (and fifty per cent following surgical menopause). Lower testosterone causes lower libido, decreased sexual desire, low mood and lower energy.

Early and premature menopause

It is good to know your menstrual cycle because it provides helpful information regarding the health and function of your ovaries, fertility and general health. There are many things that can disrupt our menstrual cycles and stop our ovaries from working before the age of 'natural' menopause, at around fifty-one. A disruption to the menstrual cycle before then is a serious issue because of its impact upon fertility and health.

Fertility changes naturally as we age and is highest in our early twenties. The chances of pregnancy reduce by the mid-thirties, as egg quality and quantity are reduced, and this lower fertility is the reason many women in that age group have issues becoming pregnant. By age forty the chances of conception per cycle is as low as five per cent, and some women may be in peri-menopause without even knowing it.

Because fertility is so precious, diagnosis of premature or early menopause is made after only four months of missed periods. The symptom of no periods is called amenorrhea, and diagnosis requires a careful history and thorough medical review. Information required includes medical treatments such as chemotherapy and radiotherapy, and specific questions to rule out polycystic ovarian syndrome (PCOS), other hormone disruptions and other medical conditions. The more questions the better the examination, and the interview is usually followed by a medical examination including blood tests.

Medical intervention, such as treatment for ovarian cancer, or as a preventative measure to reduce breast cancer risk, can cause early or premature menopause. It may involve surgical removal of the ovaries or drug treatment to stop the ovaries from functioning. Chemotherapy or pelvic radiation treatment for cancer may also reduce fertility and cause early menopause, as it may damage the ovaries. Not all chemotherapy drugs have the same risks, and for some the damage may be temporary, and age, health, drug type and dose level all make a difference. If you are wanting to protect your fertility and are undergoing treatment, please discuss this with your specialist.

The cause of naturally occurring premature menopause, as opposed to medical, remains a mystery in most cases. The loss of periods may be a symptom of a bigger health condition or genetic issue such as Fragile X syndrome and Turner syndrome, which can cause follicle depletion. Other conditions may include auto-immune diseases, metabolic disorders, and infections such as mumps or HIV. Regardless of cause, premature menopause is due to either follicle dysfunction as eggs are not released, or follicle depletion as there are no eggs left. This is very different from other conditions such as anorexia nervosa, which cause a loss of menses due to severe weight loss but not loss of eggs. However, due to the lack of understanding regarding peri-menopause and early and premature menopause, it is easy to experience threats to fertility and/or undergo peri-menopause without really knowing it.

Science bite: Medical menopause

Medical menopause is induced menopause to treat or manage a severe medical problem like breast or uterine cancers. Medical menopause is more severe than natural menopause and has increased risk of osteoporosis, heart disease, depression and anxiety, and premature death. It may involve surgical removal of the ovaries, a procedure termed an oophorectomy. Periods will stop immediately and there is the total loss of fertility, with menopause commencing immediately.

A hysterectomy is the removal of the uterus, which ends the chance of future pregnancy, but does not necessarily mean menopause. A hysterectomy may or may not include removal of one or both ovaries. In general women who have hysterectomies go into menopause four years earlier than natural age. Both surgeries are significant medical procedures and have their own risks and may also cause great grief and loss of identity.

Pharmacological menopause involves taking specific medication that stops the ovaries from making oestrogen and is linked to multiple side effects, including dizziness, nausea, blurry vision and headaches, often due to changes in blood pressure, along with stiff joints and other menopause symptoms.

Case study: Mystery unravelled

For what my doctors in the UK deemed as unexplainable, I now know the answer: peri-menopause.

Twice a day for six years, I stuck a needle in my hip and pushed the plunger down, releasing oestrogen, the potential cure for my infertility. I started down this path at age thirty-five. Who would have thought it was premature menopause? Not them and certainly not me.

After many unsuccessful rounds of treatment, including three donor egg implants, my body gave out. So along with their sympathy, I was given the talk about what might happen physically over the three-month fertility treatment detox period: irregular periods, joint pain, headaches, sleeplessness and hot flushes. I experienced those side effects in abundance except hot flushes, with only two memorable episodes.

Fast forward two years and I was done. In post-menopause there were no more red crosses on the calendar, no more late-night runs to the store for 'lady products', no more cramps, and no more hope for a child from my body.

I remember my first period at age thirteen: it was a quiet affair, it just happened without fanfare. I can say the same of my last period – it just happened, without the hot flushes, mood swings and sleeplessness. It was a quiet affair and the transition evidently began before I had even begun trying to have children.

A diagnosis of early or premature menopause can be devastating, so it is crucial to care for your physical and mental health after a diagnosis. Thankfully neither are very common. Early menopause impacts only eight to ten per cent of women, while premature menopause is rarer, affecting one per cent of women under age forty, and one in a thousand under thirty. But that still adds up to a lot of women.

In addition to the obvious fertility issues, women who experience premature and early menopause are at a much higher risk of death (all-cause mortality) compared to women who go through natural menopause at normal age. Women with menopause occurring before forty-five are at increased risk of premature cardiovascular disease, Parkinson's disease, cognitive decline, depression, anxiety, sexual dysfunction, body changes and earlier aging. There are also the significant psychological issues of loss associated with infertility, identity and purpose, as well as feelings of isolation from being out-of-step with your peers.

Treatment usually involves hormone therapy (HT) to keep hormone levels at a natural level until the time of natural menopause, to reduce the risks for cardiovascular disease and osteoporosis, and to support brain health. Therefore, many women with early or premature menopause are prescribed HT, previously known as hormone replacement therapy (HRT), until the age of fifty.

However, HT, especially when commenced at an earlier age or used for a long period of time, is not without its own consequences. The increased risk for breast cancer the longer HT is used is a real concern for many women, and the woman in the case study above developed breast cancer in her late fifties. There is a lack of good-quality information specifically examining HT use in women under the age of fifty, so it is difficult to balance the pros and cons and decide about treatment. The evidence to support taking HT for cardiovascular health, and weighing up the unknown breast cancer risk, is more obvious. Women who go through menopause before age thirty-five are three times more likely to develop heart disease than those who go through menopause at the average age, but the use of HT appears to reduce the risk compared to those who do not take it. There will be plenty of things to discuss (heart health versus breast cancer for one) with health professionals, along with partners and family.

Case study: Abrupt end

We were having difficulty getting pregnant. After the second year we had a medical review and were told my husband had fertility issues and that IVF would be our best option. I did all the injections and egg farming, which was a hormone nightmare, and pretty hard juggling with work. It took twenty-four rounds of IVF before we were blessed with twins.

Motherhood started out well, but I noticed I was tired, I had trouble sleeping and I was getting really emotional. At first, I was told it was due to my not managing the demands of parenting and my return to work, too much stress – all of which made me feel like a failure and guilty. My mood swings were getting really bad and I was probably getting depressed, so I was finally referred to a psychologist.

I was asked the usual questions, including medical history, and did I have post-natal depression. When I said I'd had IVF the psychologist just stopped, asked my age, and if I knew where I was in menopause. I was shocked – it had never crossed my mind. She asked me to get it investigated and told me that IVF can bring forward menopause.

She was right. I was in early menopause at forty-three. Why didn't the doctors tell me? Instead they had judged me.

Early and premature menopause have unique challenges, therefore it is vital for women to be proactive and receive medical attention as soon as symptoms of hormone changes become evident. It is advisable to adopt appropriate self-care strategies and a healthy lifestyle to protect optimal health and reduce further health risks. Additionally, look after your mental health and remain connected to others who make you feel positive, as those who experience early or premature menopause often have more menopause symptoms and a more difficult transition experience.

Self-care: Maximise wellbeing in early and premature menopause

- **Investigate.** As soon as your periods stop, or dramatically change, start monitoring. Take a pregnancy test. Test your hormone levels and arrange a thorough medical examination and differential diagnosis if you miss periods or they change dramatically – especially if you are under age forty.
- **Manage fertility.** Get a referral to a fertility clinic if you want to or think you might want to have children in the future. And also arrange contraception, because you never really know for sure if there is an egg or not being released, and HT is not protective.
- **Protect your body.** Address all your physical health needs and manage the risks associated with early or premature menopause. There is no treatment for premature menopause so arrange the best medical management you can for bone protection and cardiovascular health.
- **Consider HT.** Give your body the hormones it requires until the time of natural menopause to prevent health issues and disease risks associated with loss of oestrogen, such as osteoporosis and cardiovascular disease.
- **Be informed.** Ask questions and seek accurate information regarding your body, fertility, treatment and any other medical procedures.

- **Connect.** Talk to supportive people, and those who can help you process all your emotions. Build your support network as necessary and consider joining relevant social support groups or online communities.
- **Reflect.** This is a big change in your life plan, whether you planned to have children or not. You may need to grieve and adjust your goals and plans – but remember that many dreams can still be achieved, if perhaps in a different way. Take the time to reflect on yourself and your needs and set new goals if necessary.
- **Seek professional help.** If you are feeling overwhelmed by distress or by strong difficult emotions, contact your treating health professional or seek psychological help.

Body changes

Apart from your ovaries changing hormone production during the menopause transition, there are multiple changes going on. In fact, some of the changes start when periods are still relatively regular. Initially your body must accommodate the rapidly changing cocktail of oestrogen and progesterone during peri-menopause and then the gradual depletion. This cannot be repeated enough: your body will manage and adapt, and you can help it along by taking good care of your health and wellbeing.

Age is important in the menopause transition as it takes place when we enter midlife, the central period of the lifespan. Aside from menopause, midlife has its own health changes, and poor health and lifestyle choices in younger years also start to affect the body and aging process. For example, as we age inflammation and oxidant levels increase, leaving us more vulnerable to a whole variety of age-related changes and diseases. If we have misused alcohol and drugs, smoked cigarettes or had a poor diet they will be even worse. Then we enter the menopause transition and the drop in oestrogen further increases the levels of oxidative stress and inflammatory cytokines in the body, aging us still further. Because the human lifespan has extended so much, we are learning much more about the effects of menopause, and the effects of age, and sometimes it is hard to separate them out.

Get a big-picture view of the menopause transition so you can best manage the changes you experience and maintain your quality of life. As I've said before, the menopause journey is very individual, even though half of humans complete it! Therefore, relying on the advice and experience of others can be helpful, but it might not always accurately fit your experience or health needs. It will be more helpful to reflect on your own situation and symptoms to develop your own roadmap through this hormone journey.

Science bite: Summary of key oestrogen functions in the body

- Maintains blood vessels and vascular health
- Supports skin function, texture and hydration
- Retains salt and water for hydration and fluid balance in the body
- Increases bone strength and calcium for bone heatlh
- Decreases cortisol and stress responding
- Helps manage gastrointestinal track by improving smooth muscle function in the intestines and stomach, reduces bowel motility and increases cholesterol in bile
- Promotes lung function by supporting alveoli
- Assists thyroid function
- Regulates immune function
- Increases platelet adhesion and supports coagulation so our blood can clot bleeds

---

Hot flushes and night sweats

Hot flushes are the most commonly reported symptom of the menopausal transition and are experienced by about seventy per cent of all women. Depending upon where you live they are also called hot flashes. Flashes is perhaps more apt as they are so sudden and there is no subtle flush but instead a hot fire! The American term 'power surge' is also becoming increasingly popular, with its positive connotations. All these terms reflect a sudden feeling of surging heat or warmth, usually starting over the chest and moving up to the neck and face. Although they can be as low impact as occasional, short, subtle rushes of heat, they can nevertheless be very frequent and quite overwhelming and may considerably compromise quality of life. For many women, they are also the most inconvenient, uncomfortable and disruptive symptom of the whole transition. They start in peri-menopause and continue in menopause.

When hot flushes occur at night they are termed night sweats, and they ruin sleep. I know a gorgeous woman who is an avid swimmer. The first night sweat she had happened when she was dreaming she was swimming, only to wake hot and to find a pool of sweat on her chest! Whether it was the dream, the heat or the pool that woke her, finding yourself awake when you need to be asleep can become a serious problem.

Case study: Still hot

It is hard to remember when menopause started, my mid-fifties I think, and I am seventy-six now. It was always at night in bed that I noticed. I would start feeling really hot and sweaty. I would pull off the bedclothes and put my feet out and after a while the heat would go away.

I remember thinking, I will get over this. I was on HRT for possibly eight years and ceased sometime after 2003, as there was a scare about being on for too long. I thought I'd come off HRT and had thought my menopause was over, but it wasn't the case. The flushes returned.

Now the flushes are almost gone. I am healthy and have always had a balanced weight and exercise more now than any other time in my life. I still have hot flushes but to a lesser extent. They mainly happen in the hotter weather. I still take off the covers and put my feet out.

The cause of hot flushes is still a bit of a mystery, but the best explanation is that the fluctuation and reduction of oestrogen upsets the brain's regulation of body temperature. We know that the decline in oestrogen disrupts the function of the hypothalamus, part of the brain that produces many hormones to regulate many body functions, including those that manage body temperature. Its job is to maintain our body heat within a specific range, but, because of the hormonal disturbance of menopause, the range of acceptable temperatures becomes too narrow. As a result, the hypothalamus often thinks the body is overheated and wants to cool the body down when in fact the body is still at a healthy temperature. For example, have a hot drink or eat chilli and garlic, and your body temperature will rise slightly and that is not a problem. But when the hypothalamus becomes more sensitive to – or less tolerant of – these subtle temperature changes during menopause it overreacts.

The problem is that to cool down our inner or core temperature we will initially feel hotter. The heart beats faster to increase blood flow to the skin and causes blood vessels to dilate to help get rid of the heat. This sudden increase in blood flow brings with it more heat, and warm blood near the surface means skin temperature can rise several degrees and we often go red as well. It also triggers sweating, which is the body's response to cool itself down. First the sweat cools you down and then as it evaporates some heat is removed. The problem is that the brain's misjudgement of excessive body heat also sends out an alert signal and the stress response is activated, which can lead to feelings of dread or anxiety during the flush, and some women even experience an aura (see page 93).

Hot flushes usually come on suddenly, but, like migraines, they may be preceded by symptoms such as increased heart rate or having prickly or tingly skin. This warning may provide enough time to allow you to take off a layer of clothes, get an ice pack or towel, get out your fan, undo a button or two or untuck a top. The flush when it happens is an extreme sense of heat surging upwards from the chest region to face. The metabolic rate temporarily increases and during this flush, and some women also report feeling panicked, dizzy, light-headed, anxious or disconnected, and sweaty. A flush can last a few seconds to ten minutes.

One ongoing bias arising from the historical view of women's health is a belief that western women are less able to cope with their menopause symptoms than women in other countries. On this basis, a study was undertaken to determine if the number of hot flushes and night sweats women experienced during menopause varied between nations or cultures and ethnicities. Sixty-six studies were identified from North and South America, Europe, Asia, Australia and Africa – women of the world. The study found that women got hot flushes in every country, or region, and at the same rate. What a surprise. More importantly, though, the study found that other factors, not related to country, ethnicity or culture, were involved in hot flushes, such as age, diet, climate, stress level and lifestyle. Some of these factors are driven by country, ethnicity or culture but have nothing to do with female neuroticism.

For many women, hot flushes are quite debilitating. But alongside the symptom itself is the embarrassment, social discomfort or loss of 'professional' or 'public' demeanour that the hot flush can cause. For one woman, a senior executive, sitting at a board meeting and experiencing a hot flush was a disaster. Her becoming flushed, hot and sweating was interpreted as her being nervous, and the inference was that she was uncomfortable and out of her depth at such a senior level – this prompted her to take an early retirement. It would have been far more liberating for her to just tell the board, 'I am in menopause and having a hot flush,' and then she could recover and get on with the job once it passed, and ultimately this could have extended her career.

Although the precise cause of hot flushes and night sweats remains uncertain, there is a lot of evidence that lifestyle makes a big difference to their frequency and intensity. There are many things in our daily lives that can increase our temperature and thereby disrupt our internal thermostat. Just think about what happens when you open the oven door, enter a hot room, eat garlic or drink excessive alcohol – your body temperature goes up. Stress is another culprit as it increases adrenaline and cortisol, which increase heat and heart rate. Stress also reduces the ability for your adrenals to make androgens, which get converted into oestrone. Additionally, stress negatively impacts serotonin levels, and there is some understanding that serotonin may also impact hot flushes. Taken together, this suggests stress has three potential pathways to increase hot flushes, making stress reduction even more important (see Part 4). Limiting your exposure to heat variations and keeping your body temperature as even as possible, being healthy, having a positive accepting attitude and managing stress will reduce flushes and sweats.

Science bite: Weight gain

Excess weight increases the frequency and severity of flushes and night sweats and can complicate other symptoms too. Some small weight gain is natural in menopause as changing hormones affect your body composition, with the primary change being the loss of the female waist to hip curve due to increased fat accumulation around the abdomen. This happens even if diet and exercise regimes do not change. This fat shift has major health implications including increased risk of cardiovascular disease and cancer.

Self-care: Turn down the heat

- **Keep a diary.** Write down when the flushes and sweats occur – document what you are doing, eating, drinking, feeling, wearing, when each hot flush begins, as you might find a pattern or identify triggers that you can then manage.
- **Reduce the heat.** Eat fewer heat-inducing foods such as curries or foods high in garlic, chilli and ginger. Reduce sugar. Also reduce heat in the external environment – watch heating levels in winter, especially overly warm bedding.
- **Remove stimulants.** Alcohol, caffeine, cigarettes and drugs will all zoom you up and increase flush risk. For example, as your body processes alcohol at night your temperature increases. Caffeine – coffee and cola – stimulates the stress response, which impacts the vascular system and makes you hot. Cigarettes increase flushes because of the impact nicotine has on the vascular system.

- **Watch your weight.** Being excessively overweight can disrupt temperature, but equally do not get too thin either, because you need some fat to make and store oestrone. Ask your health provider for weight guidance if necessary.
- **Dress for success.** Wear clothes that can aid air flow, such as clothes without waist bands or belts – think dresses rather than skirts and tops – and wear things that can be opened or taken off easily, such as cardigans rather than jumpers. Try natural fibres such as cotton rather than synthetic ones, as they breathe better, and similarly try to have cotton bedclothes and bed linen.
- **Keep cool.** During the day, drink iced water, stay hydrated and drink fewer hot drinks. Avoid hot spaces – overheated rooms, saunas and spas – and keep cool by running cold water over your inner wrists or placing a cold towel on the back of your neck. Use a water spritzer on your face or use body wipes to freshen up after a flush. At night, keep an ice pack or damp towel nearby, and make sure your bedroom is ventilated and not stuffy.
- **Exercise.** Physically active women have fewer flushes and sweats – and remember it can be gentle regular exercise like walking, not a stress-inducing hard-core punishing regimen.
- **Manage stress.** Higher levels of stress are associated with more flushes. The stress response will make you hotter and amplify hot flushes. Learn to manage your stress; for strategies see Part 4.
- **Consider treatment.** There are plenty of options for hormonal treatment (see Part 6) and non-hormonal evidence-based natural remedies. In *all* circumstances tell your doctor and any other health professional

everything you are taking, because some products, natural or prescribed, can interfere with other treatments and can have nasty side effects.

- **Be positive.** Attitude is linked to symptom severity, so let's change the language. Rather than hot flush, how about using the American term 'power surge' instead. Try not to get frustrated and emotionally hot under the collar with having flushes, as it makes them worse: rather, try accepting them as a sign of health. With my medical menopause, I had about two hot flushes per hour. I took the heat out by simply accepting them.

Migraines

Women experience more headaches and migraines than men. With an increased understanding of hormones it is now understood that oestrogen and progesterone are linked to the incidence of some headaches and migraines. Children of both sexes have the same rates of headache until they reach puberty, and from then onwards females have approximately three times more headaches than males. Over women's lifetimes they have a forty-three per cent chance of having a migraine compared to only an eighteen per cent risk in men. Menstrual migraines affect almost fifty per cent of women at some stage in their life.

Case study: Three generations of hormone migraines

My daughter texted me from school saying that she felt weird, had black spots before her eyes and blurred vision. She felt confused and couldn't focus, and had numb fingers, and a massive headache with nausea. I thought that she may have a major neurological issue. When we got medical assistance our local doctor simply asked her if she was due to have a period! He smiled kindly (he has known her before she was born), and said, 'I am afraid you are having a menstrual migraine.'

Once home, loaded with analgesic and anti-nausea medications – she had vomited three times already – we darkened her room and popped her in bed. She slept for almost eight hours, had dinner and went back to sleep. She could do nothing. Her head throbbed; light made it worse. She had no more vomiting but felt generally sick and dizzy. She said she felt like she was dying.

My maternal grandmother used to have the same problem. I can very clearly remember when she had 'a headache'. We had to tiptoe around as she retired to lie down. She would spend several days in bed with her migraines. I also remember that her 'constant headaches' were negatively perceived by other family members, who showed frustration rather than empathy – they simply did not believe her and thought she put it on to get a rest.

I now understand my grandmother entirely. I never had a menstrual migraine, ever. Then I entered peri-menopause and, wow, wasn't I knocked for a six. The constant vice-like pain that throbs with movement and is wrapped in nausea. These migraines are totally brain-numbing mind fogs through which my thoughts struggle to connect. I want to retreat from everything for a couple of days. My train of thought just evaporates. I chomp through Nurofen [ibuprofen] and semi-function like a zombie through the two to three days that they last. I wish I could retire to bed too but can't because of work. Thankfully in the past year I have only had three! Bring on menopause.

Menstrual migraines occur in women who are particularly sensitive to fluctuations in their sex hormones. They usually occur two days before the start of the period, when progesterone is lowest, and/or for the first three days of bleeding when oestrogen and progesterone are both at their lowest levels, and in different ratios to each other. Headaches and migraines also co-occur with PMS. Oral contraception increases oestrogen and therefore increases the risks for headaches or migraines for some women, and in others may have the opposite effect and alleviate migraines by keeping levels of oestrogen constant.

Menstrual migraines do not necessarily go away with the menopause transition, and in some cases, as with the woman above, they *start* then. They can arise during peri-menopause when oestrogen and progesterone levels are erratic and continue into menopause, when oestrogen levels are almost non-existent. Twenty-five studies of menopause migraine led to the conclusion that the rates of women experiencing menopausal migraines were between ten and twenty-nine per cent. A huge number of the women with migraines said the attacks were debilitating, and eighty per cent reported they occurred more than once per month. Vasomotor (or blood vessel) symptoms of hot flushes and night sweats were linked to higher rates of migraine and interestingly the rates of migraine appeared higher during peri-menopause than menopause. The fact that migraines occur with different levels of hormones, such as during peri-menopause, suggests that migraine is sensitive to the *fluctuations* in hormones, particularly the ratio of oestrogen to progesterone, rather than to the total amount of hormones.

Science bite: Migraines

There are two types of migraine – those with an aura (MA) and those without (MO). An aura is a sensory disturbance and can include changes in vision such as flashes of light, blind spots, or tingling in the hands or down limbs or in the face. The aura precedes the headache by up to an hour and can continue once the head throb or pain starts. Migraines are syndromes, as they include a number of symptoms. Generally, MO migraines are characterised by headache in one side of the head with a pulsating quality, and are often aggravated by physical exercise or light, and are associated with nausea. MA migraines tend to have more transient focal neurological symptoms as well as the migrainous headache.

Post-menopause, some women continue to experience migraines because of a lack of hormones, and hormone therapy may be necessary. But HT can either increase or decrease risk of migraine. Post-menopausal HT has been found to be associated with *worsening* of migraines. The effects of several therapeutic regimens on migraines have also been investigated, leading to inconclusive results, and the use of treatment is still debated. To date, no specific preventative measures are recommended for menopausal women with migraine. Many women do, however, use HT quite effectively to reduce the severity and duration of migraines, so it is clearly an individual response.

Case study: Lost years

My menopause was horrific. I suffered such extreme migraines I had to stop working and retire from many things I enjoyed because I was totally incapacitated. For four to five days I would totally retreat and not leave my house. I would be bedridden with a throbbing head and could not keep anything down. I was even hospitalised with dehydration on several occasions. I tried HRT, but it made no difference at all. I suffered through eight years of menopause, but I have a new life now and am thankful it is over.

Self-care: Manage migraines

- **Keep a diary.** Track your migraines – when they occur, along with the time, type of food and drink consumed, hours of sleep beforehand, monthly cycle, allergies, stress, activities and anything else you think relevant. This will help inform health professionals about exactly when the migraine attacks begin so they can investigate triggers and form a diagnosis and plan treatment.
- **Watch your diet.** There are food triggers. Think about what you eat as there are many foods that can trigger migraines – chocolate, red wine, caffeine, monosodium glutamate food additives in processed and packaged foods, nitrates, which are another preservative, and aged cheese. Also try to avoid artificial sweeteners such as aspartame, over-ripe fruits and fermented products. Eat regular meals so your body and brain have a constant stable source of energy (glucose), and even consider slow-carbohydrate snacks as these have been found to be helpful pre-period.
- **Maintain hydration.** We are seventy-five per cent water. Dehydration shrinks the brain, slows information processing, contributes to headache and migraine, and leads to symptoms that look like menopause symptoms or makes them worse – joint pain, inflammation, mood disorders, brain fog, wrinkly skin and constipation ... to name only a few. Ideally drink plenty of water to remain

well hydrated, rather than sugar-laden or caffeinated drinks as these are potential triggers. If you are having flushes and sweats you will need to drink more than usual to compensate for the fluid loss.

- **Know your signs.** Learn to recognise your aura before the migraine starts – and take medication as soon as practical. Carry medication if necessary. Also take medication and effective proven natural remedies to manage migraine symptoms, such as anti-nausea treatment.

- **Learn to relax.** Make sure you are consistently getting enough sleep – seven to nine hours for adults under sixty-five. Delegate and reduce the demands on you and manage stress. Learn relaxation or meditation techniques to help you manage pain and assist with turning off the stress response (pain will trigger it even if the rest of life is ideal); this will also assist with sleep.

- **Accept that migraines happen.** You can't fight them so getting distressed or frustrated is simply burning up your precious energy and increasing your stress levels. Seek help instead. There are pharmacological options such as painkillers and HT, along with options such as acupuncture and meditation.

- **Take time out.** Do not judge yourself negatively if you need to withdraw or take time off. A thorough rest will help you cope and reduce your stress. Remove your superwoman cape – it is not a failing to rest. Be kind to yourself and support yourself to get through.

Science bite: Changes to your vision

Sometimes people get headaches from eye strain. All sensory functions decline with age as receptive sensitivity is lost. However, researchers are discovering that even our eyes have some 'sex' hormone receptors in them, though they don't really know yet what that means for function or possible changes over the menopausal transition. What we do know is that women report changes in their vision during pregnancy, menses and menopause, thus linking sex hormones and vision. In particular, changes appear to influence the equilibrium of the eye and symptoms may include blurred vision or reduced vision, tired eyes and red eyes. There are also normal age-related changes in lens length. Be vigilant regarding your eye health and keep an eye on your vision.

Sleep disturbance

After hot flushes, sleep disturbance is the second most common complaint of women going through the menopause transition. Women report more disruption to their sleep than men and their difficulties increase with age, starting from peri-menopause. A study of over sixteen thousand women found that sixteen to forty-two per cent of peri-menopausal women reported disturbed sleep whereas by menopause the number had risen to thirty-five to sixty per cent of women. Delayed sleep onset, or difficulty falling asleep, appears to be an issue for one in ten women. In contrast, difficulties staying asleep are evidently a bigger problem, affecting one in three women during peri-menopause and menopause, and the disturbance is not necessarily due to night sweats.

There are several reasons why women may experience disturbed sleep during the transition and it can be easy to immediately blame poor sleep on hormonal shifts, but it may not necessarily be the cause. Poor sleep is a very common problem and there are many factors which reduce quality and quantity of sleep. It is, therefore, important to review all possible causes of sleep disturbance.

Increasing age changes sleep. Changes to sleep patterns occur naturally across the lifespan and are a consequence of the natural aging processes in both men and women. On the other hand, poor sleep may be a symptom of poor health, high stress, mental illness, sleep disorder and/or hormonal change. Some suggest that the hormonal changes of menopause make no difference at all to sleep quality and that any sleep disturbance is all due to age.

How does age affect sleep? As we get older we naturally have less time in deep sleep and tend to wake more easily after rapid eye movement (REM) sleep. Sleep efficiency, a global objective measure of sleep achieved, apparently does not vary much due to menopause status. This is important. What this suggests is that although women might wake often, their overall total sleep is still within what would be considered normal or healthy levels. So, if you wake, try to sigh and relax and return to sleep knowing that this is normal and that you are going to be fine.

The primary causes of disturbed sleep for midlife women during the transition are in fact primary sleep disorders, including insomnia, sleep apnoea and restless legs syndrome – now referred to as Willis-Ekbom disease. Broadly speaking insomnia results in difficulty falling asleep, staying asleep, or both. Sleep apnoea is a disruption in breathing – you stop breathing momentarily and then start up again. Sleep apnoea can be due to excess weight and obesity as the airways become compressed. Rates of sleep apnoea do increase in women after menopause, but this appears most often due to their increase in weight.

Science bite: Sleep

Our natural sleep–wake cycle is part of our natural circadian rhythm regulated by the brain (suprachiasmatic nucleus and hypothalamus), which sends out hormones to induce and control sleep. The system responds to light and dark – which is why it is good to turn lights down low in the evening to promote sleep and look at natural light when you wake.

There are four different stages of sleep, collectively termed sleep architecture. The stages are categorised as rapid eye movement sleep (REM) or non-rapid eye movement sleep (NREM). Three stages are NREM: transitional sleep, light sleep and deep sleep. During deep sleep, important rest, repair and restore functions are taking place as our blood pressure has dropped, our muscles are relaxed, our heart rate drops, and our breathing rate is slow and steady. We produce more antibodies to boost our immune system, and hormones are released, especially those for growth and development as well as those necessary to balance weight and metabolism. In REM most of our dreaming occurs, and it's when the brain is most active, filing information, making connections and forming new memories. REM sleep is just under being awake and comes after deep sleep.

Sleep architecture naturally changes across the age span. With increasing age, we spend less time in deep sleep and REM, and more time in light sleep. Hormonal changes, menopause, stress, health issues and life circumstances may also rob us of more sleep.

Women who had sleep problems before the menopause transition are more likely to have sleep issues during the transition. Sleep research examining subjective sleep, which is the amount of sleep women report they have, and objective ratings of sleep duration and number of sleep cycles, indicates a mismatch. Objective ratings of poor sleep efficiency in women of middle age indicate that sleep-disordered breathing, sleep apnoea, was the issue. In contrast, subjective ratings of sleep quality were influenced by hot flushes and anxiety.

Intuitively you might think that difficulties staying asleep would be due to night sweats and hot flushes – vasomotor changes. However, the science appears contradictory as to whether it is the hot flushes and sweats that cause sleep disturbance or other factors. Now if you have woken hot and sweating it probably seems obvious – you woke due to hot sweats. However, results between studies vary. The differences between studies, and therefore the variability in advice given to women, is largely due to the different forms of sleep disturbance being examined.

Sleep is an area where several hormones and neurotransmitters get involved and they each impact on different stages of sleep. Disturbed sleep can include delayed sleep onset, waking during sleep and/or waking early. Any of these sleep disturbances upsets the regulation of the sleep hormones, and other hormones magnifying any issues.

Oestrogen and progesterone both affect the hormones involved in the sleep–wake cycle. They both influence melatonin, which is crucial for sleep onset. Progesterone also acts as a sleep-promoting hormone that soothes and sedates us, so the shifting ratio of oestrogen and progesterone during peri-menopause can unsettle sleep onset so we don't fall asleep easily or within thirty minutes of going to bed. Decreasing oestrogen and progesterone levels increase cortisol, which can also make falling and/or staying asleep difficult. High cortisol levels decrease serotonin, which can impact how we feel when we wake up as serotonin helps maintain normal mood. Menopause is linked to changes in mood due to the link between oestrogen and serotonin and the risk for depression caused by imbalances in these substances (see Part 4). The complexity leads to a chicken and egg problem as mood disorders impact sleep, poor sleep disrupts hormones, and hormone changes impact mood. Thankfully, there are multiple points for intervention, including addressing stress, improving mood, establishing sleep hygiene and improving hormone health.

A woman who is not getting enough quality sleep will become tired, which has significant knock-on effects on other body systems and exacerbates all menopause symptoms, including increased stress, increased weight, slower metabolism, lower immunity and higher cardiovascular disease risk. It is important to seek appropriate care. A recent American study found that although forty-eight per cent of women aged from mid-fifties to mid-sixties report sleep problems and are more than twice as likely to use prescription sleeping aids as pre-menopausal women, they did not voluntarily report their sleep difficulties to their treating doctor.

The important thing is to actively address the factors that may be contributing to reduced sleep quality and efficiency. Primary sleep disorders, where they exist, need to be correctly identified as such, not be attributed to the menopausal transition, and then be effectively treated. Manage health issues, reduce stress, and keep active so you get tired. Also, there is evidence to suggest that sleep quality in midlife influences sleep in late life, so try to develop good sleep hygiene now so that you can enjoy the restorative and reparative benefits for the rest of your life.

Self-care: Restore sleep hygiene

- **Make sleep a priority.** Establish a regular sleep routine and a regular sleep and wake time. That way your brain can plan to release the right hormones at the right time. During the hormone chaos of peri-menopause, a strict sleep–wake routine is essential.
- **Prepare for sleep.** Get your body ready to rest and restore. Turn off screens and blue lights, which send the brain wake-up signals, and avoid stimulants, which speed you up rather than relax and sedate you.

- **Get cool.** Body temperature must drop for sleep, but if you are having vasomotor symptoms give it some help – try having a warm shower (not a hot bath), have an iced wash cloth handy and drink ice cold water. Wear cool, natural-fibre bedclothes and have cotton sheets so your skin can breathe. Keep the room ventilated and not stuffy or overheated. Think about having layers of bedding – rather than one thick quilt or duvet; lighter blanket layering might be better.
- **Tire your body.** Being physically tired helps with sleep. Exercise during the day – but not too late, as you can over-energise yourself – so you feel tired. You could also try yoga or a warm bath to help relax your muscles.
- **Calm your brain.** Being deeply relaxed assists sleep onset and returning to sleep if you wake. Try meditation, mindfulness or progressive muscle relaxation to calm the body and slow down a racing or stressed brain. Address any mental health issues. Try sleep using sleep apps.
- **Address primary sleep disorders, such as sleep apnoea.** See your health professional as sleep is crucial to optimal physical and psychological health. Check out your overall health, be a healthy weight to reduce risks of sleep disorders and check medications that may impact sleep as a known side effect.
- **Consider sleep treatments.** Treatments could be psychological, pharmacological and/or natural. Some people use magnesium and/or herbal options and alternative over-the-counter sleep remedies. The traditional glass of milk is well known to aid sleep by increasing the release of melatonin. Alternatively, you could try acupuncture or pharmacological methods such as calmative products and prescription medications like melatonin and HT. There are plenty of options.

Bones

The media campaign promoting strong bones for health and longevity has been highly successful. We are all aware we need to maintain bone health as we age to avoid osteoporosis, but we do not necessarily understand what that means. Osteoporosis is called a silent disease because we are often unaware that our bones have become fragile. Fragility fractures may cause pain, restrict function and lead to loss of independence, and possibly premature death.

Bone loss (more specifically loss of bone mineral density, or osteoporosis) is still a major health issue, particularly in women, and especially after menopause. Oestrogen has a crucial role in supporting bone health by helping maintain mineralisation. It is estimated that almost half of all women will have a fracture at some stage, and the usual sites of fracture are hip, wrist and spine. Because of oestrogen's crucial role, oestrogen patches have been used to assist bone healing in both men and women who have had multiple or complex fractures.

Our bones are living tissue and are constantly being 'broken down' (resorption) and then 'remade' (reformation) somewhere in the body at any given time. This is how we have a constant supply of calcium in our body to support many physiological processes. Increasing age is also linked to a reduction in bone strength and solidity. When we are young and still growing, more bone is made than broken down and new bone is added, and our bones become larger, longer, heavier and stronger (denser). Peak bone formation is reached around age thirty and this is when our bones have their greatest strength and density. After age thirty there is more bone resorption than new bone formation, so gradually with normal aging there is some bone loss.

Weak bones and osteoporosis arise when there is less mineral density in the new bones than the old bones they have replaced. Osteoporosis is the condition when bones are so weakened that the risk of fracture is very high. Osteopaenia indicates that your bone density is lower than normal for your age but not quite as severe – take it as an alarm to get active. There are many lifestyle factors that increase your risk of osteoporosis, such as smoking, poor diet (resulting in lack of calcium), low weight and lack of exercise. Certain medications, particularly corticosteroids, may also result in loss of bone density, and in women menopause is another significant risk.

Oestrogen regulates the process of resorption and reformation. Changes in a woman's oestrogen levels therefore impact the process of bone development, and a lowering of oestrogen means less calcium and reduced bone density. The time of rapid bone density loss is reportedly in the few years before menopause – during peri-menopause – and this continues for up to ten years post-menopause. The rate of bone loss then slows.

Another factor impacting bone density generally, and more so in menopause, is inflammation. The reduction of oestrogen is linked to an increase in inflammatory cytokines, which are not good for the body or brain. In terms of bone health cytokines stimulate increased bone turnover – the breaking down of old bones and building of new – which ultimately leads to further bone mineral loss.

If you are concerned about your bone health, have your risk evaluated. Even if you are not concerned it is a good thing to check because most of us underestimate our risks. A mid-age friend took her mother to have her bones checked and thought she would too, only to be told her bone health was worse than her mother's! A bone health check may be as simple as completing the online World Health Organization FRAX questionnaire (Fracture Risk Assessment Tool). Medical examinations test your bone health and may involve a bone mineral density (BMD) test, which provides a quick snapshot of bone health, or for diagnosis of osteoporosis, a dual energy X-ray.

Science bite: Bones, osteoclasts and osteoblasts

Oestrogen directly impacts upon the process of resorption and reformation of bones at a cellular level by regulating osteoclasts and osteoblasts. The parathyroid gland produces parathyroid hormones (PTH), which regulate blood calcium levels. When calcium levels are low, PTH targets the skeleton (and kidneys and intestine) to trigger the release of calcium. Osteoclasts are involved in bone tissue resorption to release calcium from the bones into the blood. Osteoclasts are complex cells that have more than one nuclei and lots of mitochondria and lysosomes and secrete digestive enzymes that dissolve bone tissue. Then the building of new bones is undertaken by osteoblasts through a process of deposition. Osteoblasts respond to growth factors and mechanical stress (exercise and resistance training, for example) and commence the process of remodelling termed reformation. Osteopenia and osteoporosis are caused by the loss of bone mineral density because more calcium is being taken out than replaced.

Self-care: Strengthen bones

- **Build strong bones.** Eat a highly nutritious diet including foods high in calcium and magnesium, along with zinc, copper, vitamins C, K and B6. Try to eat dairy products – yoghurt, milk, cheese – daily, along with salmon or sardines with bones, dark leafy greens and nuts. If your dietary intake is insufficient, augment with supplements.

- **Capture the sun.** Vitamin D is essential for many body processes and is better thought of as a hormone. Vitamin D helps absorb calcium so aim to get about fifteen minutes of sunshine on your arms and/or legs each day. You can also get vitamin D from eggs and fatty fish like tuna and salmon, and it is in some fortified foods.

- **Increase your strength.** Weight bearing and resistance exercise like weight training improve bone health and help prevent osteoporosis. Walking, skipping and other 'pounding' activities, such as tennis, are also good types of exercise for bones, whereas swimming works the heart but is not weight bearing. All forms of good exercise improve metabolism and help maintain physical range and function.

- **Reduce falls risk.** Be mindful where you put your feet. Slow down on wet, slippery or uneven surfaces. Remove trip hazards like rugs, things on the floor, and clutter. Use non-slip mats in the bathroom. Wear comfortable supportive well-fitted shoes, and if you like heels make sure the higher the heel the better the fit. Make sure you can see where you are going, so turn lights on in bathrooms at night and keep hallways and traffic areas well lit. Get off ladders and stay away from edges, ledges and other high structures unless you have a safety harness.

- **Medication.** There are medications to improve bone health so check with your treating doctor. There are also many medications that have the side effect of leaching bone minerals, so always check with your health physician and make sure all your medications make sense for your age and stage in life.

Science bite: Skin and hair

Hormones affect organs and our skin is the largest organ in our body. In puberty, progestogen and androgens are involved in maintaining our skin by keeping it healthy and nourished, controlling oil and metabolising collagen. Yes, collagen, the special type of protein that keeps skin plump and supple. In menopause, as oestrogen declines there is less collagen metabolised, and a loss of elastin, so we get wrinkles, thinner skin and loss of plumpness. Other changes are increased dryness of the skin due to decrease in oils and collagen, or possibly acne as androgens increase relative to oestrogen, leading to the classic hormone acne line around the jaw line, chin and neck. You may also notice increased bruising, which is due to lower collagen. Sleep, diet and hydration make a difference from the inside out, while there are many products and procedures for the outside in.

Breasts

For many women breasts signify femaleness. Oestrogen is fundamental to breast development; they grow in puberty as part of our reproductive and sexual development and are part of our female physical experience, whether we feel positive or negative about their presence. As we age and enter the menopause transition we become increasingly aware of changes to our breasts and breast cancer risk. In Australia every year around 13,000 women are diagnosed with breast cancer, and it is suggested one woman in eight will be diagnosed with breast cancer before age eighty-five (incidence rates are highest between age sixty-five and sixty-nine). However, the vast number of women do not ever get breast cancer, and of those who do get breast cancer the majority (ninety-five per cent) will not die from the cancer. We need to keep fear in perspective.

There are also plenty of things we can do to reduce our risks. One simple thing is to undergo regular mammography to screen for breast cancer from age fifty. It used to be offered to younger women, but studies have now shown the risks are not there for most women so that the risks associated with having too many scans outweigh the benefit of screening. For those who do have known risks the recommendations are different.

Known risk factors are genetic, family history, chest radiation (hence limiting the number of breast scans), alcohol use, dense breasts, increasing age and high lifetime exposure to oestrogen. However, of all cases of women who develop breast cancer, approximately fifty per cent had no known risk factors, so obviously risk is complicated. I was one of those cases with no known risks and I developed grade-3 invasive breast cancer within eight months from my last scan. There are also different types of breast cancer depending upon the area of breast tissue they develop in and they vary by type: invasive, non-invasive and metastatic. You can develop more than one type; I had three.

Breasts are loaded with oestrogen receptors and when oestrogen is in the bloodstream the receptors soak it up and trigger cell growth – that is how the breasts grow in puberty. The problem is that after puberty the breasts continue to take up any excess oestrogen in the bloodstream and the powerful signals for growth can stimulate cancerous cell growth, and the risk increases with age due to increasing cell mutations. This is why most breast cancers develop in oestrogen receptor cells – this kind of breast cancer is often described as ER positive. The more oestrogen in the breast, the higher risk of oestrogen linking to an ER-positive cell and stimulating cancer cells to grow. This accounts for the relationship between lifetime oestrogen exposure and increased risk, and why breast cancer is more common in women who take HT and/or used the contraceptive pill as these both add extra oestrogen to the body's natural levels.

What does lifetime exposure to oestrogen mean? Based on a study of over 400,000 women, breast cancer risk increases the younger you are for your first period and the older you are for your last. Older age as you enter menopause matters, as you have had high doses of oestrogen in your body for longer. Pregnancy, contraceptive pill use and HT also make a difference to lifetime exposure. Another pathway is via breast density. Younger women have denser breasts, and this increases cancer risk by four to six times. Dense breasts also make detection with mammography more difficult, and usually an ultrasound is also taken or perhaps an MRI. With increasing age and menopause, breasts become less dense.

Your breasts can tell you a lot about your oestrogen hormone status. During peri-menopause your breasts may become sore, tender and swollen, like they were during puberty or pregnancy, because of hormone fluctuations. As oestrogen levels decrease, the shape, density, texture and size of your breasts may also change. This is due to fibrocystic changes and occurs just before your periods as well as in women taking hormone therapy.

Breasts are important for post-menopause oestrogen production. Breast tissue includes fatty tissue (adipose tissue), and the hormone aromatase is mainly made by fatty tissue and changes androgens into oestrogen. Problems only arise when there is excess oestrogen. Breast cancer profoundly changes the menopause transition as treatment involves reducing oestrogen and or blocking it, and HT to manage menopause symptoms is never an option.

Self-care: Support your breasts

Healthy oestrogen balance is crucial for breast development and breast health. There are several known risks for breast cancer, and a lot of unknowns. However, there are several things you can do to reduce your risk.

- **Know your breasts.** Look at your breasts and get used to your breast shape, feel, size and density. Monitor them for any changes and understand how they may change as your hormones fluctuate. Any lump of any size needs to be examined, and monitor redness, nipple sensitivity, itchiness, pain in the breast, chest, shoulder or neck, and swellings in the armpit.

- **Prepare for the screening.** Until a woman invents a new mammography system we must rely on the current breast masher. To reduce discomfort, schedule mammograms for the week after your period, and perhaps take some over-the-counter analgesic one or two hours beforehand to reduce pain. Arrange something nice for yourself afterwards – take a walk, sit in the sunshine, enjoy a bubble bath or perhaps buy some flowers.

- **Manage your weight.** There is a recognised link between excess weight and increased risk of breast cancer as excess body fat increases the levels of oestrogen circulating in the blood. If not breast cancer, it could be another type of cancer as five per cent of cancers are associated with excess weight, and there are thirteen more cancers specifically linked to weight, such as kidney, colon, pancreatic and uterine cancers.

- **Consider your risks.** Before commencing HT please consider your lifetime exposure to oestrogen before adding more. Were you on the contraceptive pill for a long time? Did you get your period young? Consider genetic factors and lifestyle risks such as being overweight, but also understand that in half of breast cancer cases there are no known risks.

- **Limit alcohol.** Every single serve of alcohol consumed increases cancer risk, with at least seven types of cancer

known to be caused by alcohol. Breast cancer risk
increases by twenty per cent by drinking two or more
alcoholic drinks a day.

Heart health

Cardiovascular disease is still the primary killer of men and
women. In women before the transition, the risk is lower than
men's, but the risk goes up after menopause. Oestrogen helps
maintain the health of our cardiovascular system – our heart and
blood vessels (arteries, veins and capillaries) – so it is vital to care
for your heart health as oestrogen levels decline. Compromised
cardiovascular health was the most frightening consequence of my
medical menopause. Previously, I was always fit with low blood
pressure and then, suddenly, I developed hypertension and cardiac
symptoms that required hospitalisation. I now have a cardiologist
in my cancer care team and follow all heart health advice.

Menopause does not cause cardiovascular disease, but
changes in our hormones impacts our risks. Cardiovascular
disease is a class of conditions that involves the heart and blood
vessels and includes coronary artery diseases (CAD), angina
and myocardial infarction (commonly known as a heart attack).
When the blood vessels to the heart are blocked we experience
a cardiac arrest (myocardial infarction). Blood vessels need to
be flexible and smooth, but with age they can become stiff and
blocked, much like a hose in a car engine gets clogged up and
stops being effective. There are different causes for heart disease
where the blood vessels cease to work effectively and efficiently.
There are hormone mechanisms including oestrogen, which are
not fully understood, and there are the well-known primary risks
of high cholesterol, high blood pressure, diabetes and obesity.
There are preventable lifestyle factors to reduce those risks
which include eating a healthy low-fat diet, reducing excessive

body weight, especially visceral fat (around our middle), and exercising regularly.

Heart health is possibly not something most people consider when they think of the menopause transition. However, among all the symptoms experienced during menopause, probably the most disquieting or scary one is an irregular heartbeat. This is, like everything else, due to lower oestrogen and is considered a 'normal' symptom. An irregular heartbeat when the heart beats faster or more forcefully than usual is termed cardiac arrhythmia, heart palpitations, atrial fibrillation or tachycardia. Cardiac arrhythmia is not the same as cardiovascular disease. That awareness of your heart beating or feeling like it has skipped a beat or is pounding can still cause significant alarm. (Although some people like a similar rush after a strong cup of coffee or bout of exercise.)

**Science bite: Key oestrogen functions
for cardiovascular health**

- Dilates blood vessels, thereby lowers blood pressure
- Increases good cholesterol
- Decreases platelet clotting
- Lowers fat deposits in artery walls
- Releases chemicals to keep blood flow
- Regulates insulin

Women past menopause experience a higher incidence of atrial fibrillation than men. One explanation is that the overstimulation of the sympathetic nervous system (stress response) that results from decreased oestrogen can cause irregular heartbeats and heart palpitations. The atrial fibrillation that women experience substantially increases their risk of stroke. As there are multiple things that can cause an irregular heartbeat, including medication and other medical conditions, along with stress, and because of the risk of stroke, it is important to have any irregularity investigated.

Advances in cardiovascular medicine – primarily the inclusion of women in studies – has helped us understand the protective role of oestrogen in heart function. In particular the relationship between oestrogen and cardiovascular health has been extensively studied for the potential to treat cardiovascular disease.

Multiple pathways involving oestrogen's protective role influence cardiovascular function during and after the menopause transition. Recall that oestrogen is circulating freely pre-menopause and that this supports vasomotor function – which is the constriction and dilation of blood vessels – by keeping them flexible. This benefit positively impacts heartbeat, blood vessel health and blood pressure.

Medical menopause is like menopause on steroids with accelerated impact and more intense and frequent symptoms, along with side effects on cardiovascular function. In my case, with the combination of anticancer medication and pharmacological menopause I developed acute hypertension and cardia arrythmia. My consistently low blood pressure went from around 105/80 to over 178/134. I was hospitalised; all my cancer treatment was ceased before it killed me, and my ovaries had to be removed.

Oestrogen also positively affects insulin and reduces diabetes risk, and influences metabolism including glucose and lipoprotein. It also reduces fat and plaques in the blood and assists coagulation. This means oestrogen provides additional support to heart health and the vascular system by stopping blood vessels becoming hard and blocked and stopping excessive blood loss.

All of these positive impacts alter during menopause, leaving women with reduced protection. For example, in pre-menopausal women their blood pressure is lower than after menopause as blood pressure increases by as much as 5mmHg, leading to risk of hypertension, and this risk is higher than in men. Evidence also suggests that changes in the oestrogen–androgen ratio, with lower oestrogen and increased androgens, leads to increased vasoconstrictors and endothelial, or vessel lining, dysfunction.

Another suggested pathway via which menopause increases cardiovascular disease risk for women is inflammation. The decrease in oestrogen leads to activation of the stress response system with its associated increase in oxidative stress and increased inflammation and cytokines.

Science bite: Cardiovascular disease lifestyle risk factors

High LDL (bad) cholesterol clogs vessels and can cause hypertension (high blood pressure). High blood sugars harden blood vessels (atherosclerosis), and excess weight burdens the heart, causing it to overexert itself. Hence the importance of diet – a highly nutritious diet is healthy, whereas an overly processed diet high in sugar, salts and saturated fats increases risks for cardiovascular disease, as does too much food.

Fitness levels also significantly impact upon the health of our heart and cardiovascular system. Fitness, the body's ability to utilise oxygen, is measured during exercise to determine the maximum uptake, with a high value indicating higher fitness. Lower fitness is clearly linked to higher rates of cardiovascular disease, especially in women. Conversely, high fitness is linked to lower risk and lower levels of visceral fat, lower blood lipid levels and lower blood pressure, as well as lower risk of metabolic syndrome. Exercise effectively counterbalances the other risks.

Lastly, the reduction in oestrogen during menopause results in women gaining weight around their abdomen, whereas in pre-menopause it was more likely to be around their bottoms. Menopause is associated with a five-kilogram weight increase –

even if there is no other change in lifestyle. This weight gain is a natural body response to be able to produce oestrogen in fatty tissue. However, too much fat around the middle (abdominal obesity) is a major risk factor for cardiovascular disease.

Our hormones and fat cells are part of a complex system involved in the regulation of metabolism, appetite, digestion, heat regulation and so forth. We understand pretty well the links between metabolism, body fat and insulin – and food cravings which can result. Your body will store fat to ensure it has what it needs, but take care during peri-menopause as the hormonal changes can cause imbalance in insulin levels, increasing the risk of insulin resistance and much higher weight gain. Studies show that almost thirty per cent of women aged fifty to fifty-nine are obese and the risk of obesity increases in post-menopause so excessive weight gain is a real health issue for many.

In animal studies oestrogen appears to help regulate body weight, with lower levels of oestrogen linked to higher food consumption and lower levels of physical activity. It is also suggested that reduced oestrogen slows metabolic rate, meaning the body converts more energy to stored fat. Other factors which contribute to this increased risk of weight gain include normal aging, genetic factors, physical inactivity, type II diabetes, hypertension and dyslipidaemia (too much free-floating fat in the blood). We can't change our age, but as aging is linked to a natural loss of muscle mass and increase in fat, we can target these natural processes by increasing our physical exercise, especially resistance training, which increases the rate at which the body uses energy – meaning it increases metabolism and reduces energy storage (fat). The other thing to watch is sleep, as tiredness and fatigue increase insulin, making us snack on energy-rich foods.

Post-menopausal women are generally older than pre-menopausal women and increasing age is a significant risk for cardiovascular health, so it is hard to untangle. But a huge community longitudinal study called the Lifelines Cohort study in Europe did just that. In the study age was separated from menopausal status in over 60,000 women, classified into pre-menopause, peri-menopause and post-menopause (surgical or natural) groups, for every year of age between eighteen and sixty-five. What they found was that blood pressure, body mass and bad cholesterol were all higher in post-menopausal women, and all went up with age. Therefore, menopause status and age are independently related to cardiovascular health. They also identified that women with surgical menopause had the highest risks of all, suggesting that natural menopause is gentler on the entire body or allows some adjustments so as to have lower risks. The outcome is that while age cannot be changed, women's increased risks for cardiovascular disease can't simply be dismissed as age related and women must actively address their cardiovascular risks post-menopause.

Cardiovascular disease and heart attack (myocardial infarction) are too often portrayed as diseases of men. The research until recently has also been male dominated and there are not enough studies including women around menopause and post-menopause. This has contributed to an unconscious bias in the medical profession. A 2018 Australian study demonstrated that women presenting with cardiac arrest are less likely than men to undergo diagnostic tests, treatment and referral for prevention. As a consequence women are more likely to die from heart attack than men. Even the advertising campaign for heart attack prevention and symptom recognition is very male focused, which is problematic as the symptoms men and women have are different. Women experience symptoms such as fullness in the chest, pain in the back, jaw or neck, racing heart and feelings of anxiety, or stomach cramps, not the stereotypical 'male' symptoms of pain in the left arm, cold sweats and suffocating chest pain. Know the symptoms. Actively monitor your heart health and be assertive to get necessary medical care.

Case study: Splitting heart

The advent of 'The Change' literally tore my heart. I went from fit and healthy, with a penchant for positive psychology – OK, perhaps that day I was a bit stressed – to a woman with a heart condition. It was Tuesday and one of those days that makes optimism cower. What I do remember very clearly is the neck and shoulder pain that came on at the end of the Monday night – not that unusual because I have an old whiplash injury that tends to play up. The discomfort persisted the whole of the next day, but as my son got into the car following after-school activities, I got a fright (I'd been lost in a book I was reading), leading to pain in my chest and upper back behind my chest, which really ached. Pain radiated into my neck – it felt like a blood vessel was distended. I put some arnica on it – my go-to cream when my neck aches – but it felt odd and the pain leached into my jaw, which seemed wrong. This was quite severe and my back hurt when I breathed. Nothing too untoward, but I felt a bit nauseated and I have an iron constitution. There was a feeling … I can't tell you what it was, I just felt like something was wrong.

So … I ordered my daughter into the shower and my son to bring our parrots inside, and I rang my husband to ask him to come home early so I could go to the doctor. He agreed, but after googling my symptoms, and really, I already feared the symptoms were those of a heart attack (but I do have a vivid imagination), I decided it was better to go to the doctor straight away.

I should mention that my sister had had a spontaneous coronary artery dissection (SCAD) the previous year and I was very familiar with heart attack symptoms. But I'd had loads of heart tests and been given the all clear. Besides, my sister has a bicuspid valve and I don't. I remembered her saying, if you have chest pain and systemic symptoms go to a doctor. This was more back pain and an odd sensation in my throat.

Systemic symptoms? Nausea, yes. Difficulties breathing, no, not yet. Shortness of breath … well, I was being a drama queen, I thought, but yeah, I could tick off quite a few of the heart attack symptoms so, while it seemed crazy, I piled the kids into the car, with a 'Bring your iPad, you can go on screen.' Fun times! By the time I backed out of the driveway, I thought, no, I'll go to the closest hospital, which I knew didn't have an Emergency Department, but this was urgent! We arrived, parked, got to the entrance and by then, I could tick the shortness of breath box – anxiety? – but the sign was unfriendly and advised any wannabe emergency people to go to another hospital, some ten minutes away … right, I thought. Too trained in obeying unfriendly signs, we returned to the car and I thought, I should have another ten more minutes in me. By then I was worried. I lectured my ten-year-old son about the symptoms I had and said I might need to pull over – if I do, you dial 000 and ask for an ambulance. We made it to the hospital, almost didn't make it across the busy road to the ED (which would have added another layer of complexity!), and I told the triage nurse my symptoms (a textbook list that screamed Heart Attack to me). 'Take a seat,' she said, and I turned to see a waiting room FULL of people. I found a seat and thought, Well, if this gets worse, I'm not too far from medical help. The kids were blissfully engaged playing Minecraft. If only all of life's problems could be so readily minimised.

After a few minutes, I heard my name called and a nurse asked me to repeat my breathlessly delivered list. 'Perhaps you'd better come through and lie down' – hallelujah!

'Yes,' I said, 'that would be good.' The understatement of the century! And so the kids settled onto the floor lost in Minecraft bliss, while I was wired and needled. Probably just as well they were distracted given the tests and my resistance to being given morphine. 'I'm not in that much pain,' I argued. 'I don't like to take painkillers.' 'It's heart protective,' the nurse assured me, 'and important.' 'I'm scared of it,' I answered, 'and I avoid it like the plague.' Turns out, I'm allergic to the stuff. My throat seized, and I couldn't breathe. It was by far a worse experience than the actual heart attack. An ambulance ride to a big-city hospital later, more tests and admission to the cardiac ward, and I was diagnosed with SCAD involving a forty per cent dissection of the oblique marginal vessel [a small branch of the coronary arteries].

When in later discussion with my cardiologist – yes, I did cardiac rehab and I now have to take heart meds forEVER more – he disputed the relationship between SCAD and menopause. Yet it seems SCADs are most likely to occur following the birth of a child or, you guessed it, in the lead-up to menopause.

My younger sister, by the way, had gone into early menopause!

Science bite: SCAD

Spontaneous coronary artery dissection (SCAD) presents like a heart attack but it is caused by the tearing of an artery wall. The artery walls have three layers and when a tear occurs bleeding causes a bulging on the innermost layer and obstructs blood flow to the heart muscle, which leads to heart attack. SCAD occurs most often in women who are otherwise healthy, with few or no risk

---

factors for heart disease. Some studies have pointed to a hormonal link, showing a greater incidence among post-partum women (thirty per cent) and women who are experiencing or close to a menstrual cycle. Menopause, extreme stress or exercise, and connective tissue disorders have also been associated with SCAD, but as yet it is not known exactly what causes it. SCAD is difficult to diagnose before it causes a heart attack, because it doesn't have any warning signs. And although it can cause a life-threatening coronary incident, SCAD patients don't typically have other heart disease risk factors.

Although SCAD is exceedingly rare, there are several take-home messages. First, do not panic: it is very rare and unlikely. Second, if you are experiencing symptoms of heart attack get help. If you don't *fit the profile,* be assertive and get your symptoms investigated. Third, educate doctors to consider SCAD in healthy women presenting with symptoms typically associated with heart attack, especially those without traditional cardiovascular disease risk factors.

Self-care: Help your heart

- **Watch your weight.** There is a natural tendency to put on weight with age and menopause, so keep within a stable healthy weight range. Not too heavy and not too light. If necessary, lose excess weight as medically advised.
- **Eat a heart-healthy diet.** Eat healthy, nutritious, slow-energy-release foods (those with a low glycaemic number) to keep energy and insulin levels in balance as well as maintain complete health and wellbeing. Limit unhealthy fats, which clog blood vessels, and excessive sugar, which hardens them.

- **Keep physically fit.** Increase your exercise level and make it a regular habit. Brisk walking so you can't sing and walk at the same time is sufficient to give your heart a workout. If possible, try to include resistance training, which will boost metabolic rate and increase your aerobic exercise to improve your heart health.
- **Reduce salt.** Excessive salt is a major health risk to our entire body. Salt increases water retention, which increases blood pressure, which burdens the heart. It also strains the brain and kidneys and increases risk of heart attack, strokes and dementia.
- **Cease cigarettes.** Chemicals in tobacco smoke cause the blood to thicken and form clots inside veins and arteries. This damages blood vessels and increases risk of atherosclerosis, stroke and heart attack.
- **Limit alcohol.** Alcohol in high amounts leads to hypertension – raised blood pressure – which causes the heart to work harder.
- **Monitor and manage your health.** Have medical check-ups as required or suggested by your treating health professionals to monitor cholesterol and blood pressure so you can reduce atherosclerosis risk and maintain optimal heart health.

Summary: Optimising menopause body health

We all know we need to invest in our health for optimal wellbeing yet, all too often, we neglect this as the demands of daily life take over. Life and everything in it is much easier to manage and enjoy from a position of health. Lifestyle plays a significant role in keeping our physical age the same as our chronological age.

Menopause is a great opportunity to put the brakes on unhealthy habits and to develop health-enhancing ones. To build optimal health consider addressing these basic foundations so you are in the best position to manage and cope with your menopause journey.

While hormone therapy is always an option, another consideration is to address each hormone-related symptom directly rather than increasing hormones per se. For example, target sleep by adopting good sleep hygiene, manage stress during the day, learn meditation, implement healthy habits and augment with herbs or medication to help sleep.

- **Prioritise your health.** Make menopause the time to transform your health today as well as starting to invest in your future. If you do not care for yourself, you risk letting down those who rely on you and limiting your ability to thrive in your next decades.
- **Restore sleep.** Lack of restorative sleep increases stress, weight gain and hot flushes, and reduces immune function, heart health and hormone balance. Prioritise sleep by aiming for a regular pattern of between seven and nine hours every night. Prepare for sleep by having a regular sleep routine and prepare to stay asleep by reducing intrusions such as gadget interruptions, toileting, getting too hot, excess light, pets and people.
- **Choose nutritious food.** A healthy nutritious diet is not medicine, but it will keep you healthy and energised and reduce disease risks, as well as support every bodily function, your brain and your mental health. Eat every four to five hours during the day; include protein, slow carbohydrates, one or two pieces or fruit and plenty of vegetables. Get enough calcium and magnesium and limit foods that rock the balance and increase stress and hot flushes, such as alcohol, chilli, garlic and caffeine.

- **Manage your stress load.** High chronic stress increases hot flushes, disease risks, weight gain, sleep disturbance and mental illness, and impacts your brain function. Learn to manage stress – reduce physiological stress by eating well, getting enough sleep regularly, and addressing pain and health issues. Reduce psychological stress by learning to say no, problem solving, delegating and changing your mindset.
- **Keep at an ideal weight.** Being too fat or too thin is not healthy, so try to get into your ideal weight range and stay there. Excess weight, especially around the internal organs, is a significant issue. Excess fat increases oestrogen and throws out many hormones in ways that increase disease risks including diabetes, thirteen types of cancer, and cardiovascular disease.
- **Move.** Exercise, and not sitting for hours, is fundamental to human health. Exercise helps manage our sleep–wake cycle, reduces stress and dementia risk, and boosts hormone function, bone health and cardiovascular health as well as our brain and mental health. The recommendations are for at least two and a half hours per week, ideally a little every day and including both resistance training and aerobic exercise.

More detailed and additional strategies are provided at the end of each part.

PART 4

MENOPAUSAL BRAIN AND MIND

Menopause impacts all our organs including the gorgeous one between our ears – the female brain. Keeping a clear head and a calm mind during the transition can be a challenge as sex hormones affect how the brain develops, operates and performs cognitive and emotional processes as well as motivating behaviour. Many women report forgetfulness, losing words and brain fog. Brain fog is not a diagnostic term but a perfect description of feeling hazy and an easily recognisable symptom. Brain fog is something some women may have experienced during pregnancy, another time of significant hormonal upheaval, and like then it will pass. However, for some women the change in their previously reliable brain due to the transition causes significant difficulties, compromising their functioning, and is a great concern to them.

Cognitive complaints are not necessarily attributed to menopause and are often linked to other menopause symptoms such as disturbed sleep, or the emotional upheaval of the transition. Many do not think that menopause is the direct cause. As a result, women may sometimes feel they are failing to manage and so doubt themselves. The consequence of concern and stress is that it increases many menopausal symptoms, such as an increase in hot flushes and further sleep disturbance. This sets a negative spiral which cumulates into greater symptom burden. Menopause affects our brains, but let's take care so it does not negatively impact our lives.

Case study: Team leader

It's very hard to work with a foggy brain. When you're a person who works a lot and is organised, busy and efficient and then you turn into a jumbled person it's hard. Some days I can't go through my to-do list and get things done, and work suffers. If you work closely with others it is important to let them know. Menopause is not a shameful thing. With my team I tell them 'I've got menopause brain today' when I get muddled. I get disorganised and do things the wrong way and slower. I feel uncoordinated in my brain. When I can, I go somewhere and sit quietly and relax to clear my head. Some days everything takes twice as long – I am just not as efficient, and I have to let them know. I just have to say, 'Bear with me. I will get there in the long run.'

One of my team (a male) bought me a hand fan because of my hot flushes which I laughed about but really appreciated. I have to communicate with family too. I've got two daughters, they are women themselves now, aged twenty-nine and thirty-two, and I find that their lack of understanding is a problem. They say, 'What's your problem?' or 'What is wrong with you?' They just think Mum is having an off day. So I do get stressed from that, and one works with me and she gets impatient and intolerant and that makes things worse. They all forget, or don't really understand, so I have to keep reminding them – telling them when I am having a menopause brain day.

Oestrogen, the brain and cognition

Oestrogen is an essential brain player, maintaining brain health and function throughout the entire lifespan. It has a direct role in prenatal development, growth in puberty and hormonal changes throughout adulthood, including menopause and old age. Oestrogen also regulates neuronal biochemistry, structure and function related to cognitive and emotional processes.

Oestrogen is widely used throughout the brain by brain cells (neurons), the support cells in the brain called astrocytes, and to maintain brain-tissue-specific functions. There are oestrogen receptors in some brain cells in specific areas of the brain. This means that oestrogen is required for them to function – imagine oestrogen as a key in a lock that turns things in the brain on. In all these areas, oestrogen has been described as neuroprotective because of its brain-benefiting roles.

Brain health is protected by oestrogen because it assists brain cell communication. An area where this is especially important is the cholinergic system, which is involved in learning and memory. Oestrogen increases the production of two important neurotransmitters (acetylcholine and glutamate) that help memory processing and learning – which is the process of encoding or developing new memories. The link between oestrogen and memory explains why some women report forgetting and memory difficulties during menopause, as low oestrogen levels mean the brain does not have enough of the essential ingredients to make new memories. The difficulty is not forgetting per se, but rather not making the memory in the first place.

Oestrogen also helps protective functions in the brain, such as reducing free radicals and influencing genes that control how neurons adapt, regenerate and grow – a process of dynamic change termed neuroplasticity. When we learn new things, such as a new language or how to operate a new television remote, our brain makes changes. Keeping our brain stimulated and challenged leads to brain growth and builds brain reserve, which makes the brain resilient. In this way, oestrogen helps protect the brain by helping it to be neuroplastic.

It is now understood that the brain produces some oestrogen itself because this hormone is so crucial to its health. Specifically, the brain's hypothalamus produces oestradiol – the same type of oestrogen produced by the ovaries – so that it has its own independent supply. Animal studies indicate that when oestradiol levels circulating in the blood are low the hypothalamus begins production to maintain the brain's crucial supply of oestrogen. When levels of our sex hormones are changing, as they do during puberty, pregnancy and menopause, the brain oestrogen receptor cells are not able to operate in the same way. This neuro-oestradiol therefore buffers the brain for changes or fluctuations in the levels of circulating oestrogen and ensures that brain health is maintained. The brain can continue to function when the ovaries are inactive, as they are before puberty and in menopause.

Science bite: Oestrogen and the brain

Research investigating oestrogen (oestradiol, or E_2) and the central nervous system has been limited because previous studies used male rodents. Overall, the molecular and neuroanatomical targets of oestrogen require further investigation. What preliminary findings show is that the action of oestrogen in the brain is controlled by two receptor systems – one for sexual reproduction and behaviour, and the other for brain function – and that the oestrogen receptor sites in the brain are not evenly distributed – meaning they are site specific. E_2 regulates the amount and function of monoamines (neurotransmitters like serotonin), neurogenesis (the development of new brain cells), inflammatory processes, and the cholinergic system used in cognition and emotional function. The oestrogen receptors have also been identified as influencing other hormones including vasopressin, oxytocin and prolactin-containing neurons

---

in the hypothalamus, and the corticosterone response to stress. The role of oestrogen receptors in brain tissue remains unknown and the discovery that oestrogen is localised in the cell nucleus of some brain cells and impacts DNA binding is hugely significant, as it suggests that oestrogen may possibly play a role in our genetic material – specifically, that oestrogen may impact the telomeres of our genes and therefore influence how well our body ages.

If oestrogen impacts brain processes and metabolism, it follows that it will influence cognition. Our various mental processes are termed cognitive functions and include such things as memory, problem solving, information processing, reaction time, language and emotional regulation. Animal studies have confirmed that oestrogen is very important for cognitive function. In studies of female rodents where their ovaries have been removed, certain cognitive tasks become much more difficult for them to complete than was the case before surgery. The cognitive difficulties experienced involve memory. Rodents are given tasks that involve learning and remembering how to find food in a maze or remembering where to find a resting platform in a water tank. After they have had their ovaries removed the rats can't find the food or water platform. Their difficulties with memory function match the findings that oestrogen influences the neurotransmitters used in processing memory and learning. Importantly, the results confirm what many women already know – that during menopause, when there is limited oestrogen, remembering anything becomes difficult.

When women during peri-menopause and menopause complete neuropsychological testing there are consistent mild difficulties in the specific cognitive domains of memory and learning, and verbal fluency. These domains match those areas where brain and functional differences are noted in development between biological females and males, and where oestrogen receptors are located. Additionally, cognitive functions requiring sustained concentration and effort also suffer, especially when there is mental confusion and cognitive fatigue.

A recent study of over two hundred women in post-menopause examined the relationship between hormone levels and cognitive function. The women were randomly grouped to receive either oestrogen, testosterone or nothing for one month. Cognitive testing indicated that spatial ability, verbal fluency and memory performances were different depending upon group allocation, meaning that oestrogen and testosterone levels both alter brain function. The fact that things changed during one month highlights the powerful influence hormones have on our brain and cognition, and hints at how significant the impact will be over a lifetime.

Stage and age at onset of menopause appear to make a difference to the extent of cognitive difficulties. Recent research also indicates that young age at onset of menopause is associated with more significant cognitive difficulties. Greater memory difficulties are also experienced during the initial phase of menopause because alternative sources of oestrogen production have not been fully developed. It is also widely accepted that surgical or medical menopause causes cognitive difficulties because it is so sudden and the body and brain have not been able to gradually adapt. In contrast, some debate remains as to whether natural menopause leads to any cognitive differences despite recent evidence.

One comprehensive study of over eight hundred women experiencing natural menopause examined oestrogen and cognitive function in late life and oestrogen exposure over the whole lifespan. They recorded all those life stages that increase or decrease oestrogen levels in women, such as age at first period, length of time taking oral contraceptives, number of pregnancies, and onset of menopause. The results indicated that each of these major hormonal phases in a woman's life influenced cognitive function including global cognition and specific cognitive domains of verbal fluency, executive function and memory. Higher lifetime exposure to sex hormones, from early onset of periods (before age eleven), older age at pregnancy, late onset of menopause, and long-term use of oral contraception, improved cognitive function. You will probably count your oestrogen exposure now like I did. I was late to start periods, took oral contraception for only five years, had two pregnancies at ages twenty-nine and thirty, and medical menopause at fifty – placing me at the lower end of total oestrogen exposure. That did not stop me from getting oestrogen-driven breast cancer, but perhaps explains why my medical menopause was earlier than my brain desired and caused so much havoc. Thankfully, there are other significant factors that influence brain health and cognition, and we have control over many of them. The other good news is research suggests that as the length of time post-menopause progresses, memory difficulties are reported less and less frequently.

Science bite: Monthly brain changes

Cutting-edge research suggests that our sex hormones may change our brain structure monthly with our menstrual cycle. Brain-imaging technology has enabled researchers to examine subtle changes in the circuits involved in learning and memory formation during the menstrual cycle. When women have increased oestrogen during their menstrual cycle their memory improves. Examination of the hippocampi (two structures crucial for memory and learning) revealed that oestrogen increases the connectivity between brain cells in the hippocampi by as much as twenty-five per cent. A more recent investigation in 2016 into premenstrual mood scanned the brain of the same women for four menstrual cycles and found that hippocampal volume increased and decreased in size with each cycle. As

---

oestrogen levels rose the volume of the hippocampi also rose due to increased grey and white matter, and then as oestrogen levels fell the hippocampi declined in a beautiful rhythm. Animal studies have confirmed the changes only occur in females and not males. Human studies also found that women's decision making was improved (and less impulsive) with higher levels of oestrogen. Low oestrogen at the beginning of a menstrual cycle also had positive benefits, as greater brain activity when thinking about positive experiences has been identified. The study authors hypothesised that the dynamic fluctuations may have developed to enable stable brain function and behaviour as protection against the cyclical changes in hormones necessary for menstruation. Essentially, brain changes occur so that women can maintain fertility without losing their cognitive function. These changes are clearly adaptive and theoretically counter any negative impacts of high or low oestrogen levels.

Menopause, memory and dementia

As previously reported, oestrogen influences memory and the brain structures associated with memory. Low levels of oestrogen mean low levels of specific neurotransmitters required for memory formation, which reduces the amount of information transfer and consolidation. Since oestrogen impacts memory, the links to cognitive decline and dementia are unavoidable. Do not panic. The links between oestrogen and dementia are complex and largely inconclusive. Dementia is certainly a terrifying prospect but having cognitive changes during menopause is not the same as having dementia. The cognitive changes associated with menopause are most likely just part of the transition, which is temporary, deterioration rarely continues a downward trajectory, and the difficulties are not usually so severe as to constitute an impairment.

You may recall at the beginning of this book I referred to women who were worried they had early dementia because of their poor memory, not realising that it might simply be menopause. Menopause memory changes are temporary and not severe. The difference between menopause and dementia comes down to cause.

Increasing age is the greatest risk factor for dementia. Women have a higher risk of dementia than men. We also live longer. Lifestyle factors play a significant part in our late-life brain health and possibly account for up to two out of three cases of dementia. For example, smoking and a lack of physical exercise significantly contribute to dementia risk and may account for up to as much as twenty-five per cent of it. There are also hormonal factors, but their role is small by comparison to the lifestyle risks, and there is not a substantial body of research on the role of oestrogen in dementia specifically at this time.

When we enter menopause we are getting older. The brain naturally undergoes age-related changes, so it can be tricky to isolate which changes are caused by age and which may be due to menopausal hormonal changes. Some functions such as our general knowledge and vocabulary in fact continue to steadily increase as we get older. Other cognitive functions – for example, memory, reaction time and thinking speed – naturally decline. 'Age-related cognitive decline' refers to changes in cognition normally occurring with increasing age, much as visual acuity also naturally deteriorates with advancing age. Such changes are normal and occur in both men and women, and there is a huge amount of individual variability. The other important fact is that the brain changes linked to dementia start decades before symptoms are evident – which means they may start *before* menopause, when our hormone levels are high. This is why it is crucial that we adopt healthy habits and take control over the lifestyle-related factors now as they influence our brain health and how we age in future.

Case study: Terrified

I recognise some changes in myself and I'm not sure I can change them. I had a total hysterectomy in 2013 and they took my ovaries. My memory has got progressively worse since then. I was fifty-three. I am really concerned about my memory, in particular remembering spoken words and conversations. My mother had vascular dementia, so I think I am getting it too. I have this fear I have got something [neurological] as I just can't keep up at work any more.

Science bite: Oestrogen and memory formation

Oestrogen decline leads to lower levels of enzymes necessary for mememory. Choline acetyltransferase is an enzyme required for the synthesis of acetylcholine, a neurotransmitter associated with memory function. Specifically, with lower levels of acetylcholine the nerve cells in the hippocampal memory structures have fewer spines for communication, which means less information transfer in memory. A reduction of acetyltransferase is found in humans diagnosed with Alzheimer's disease. In rodents the introduction of oestrogen replacement leads to an increase in the hippocampal spine numbers so that the numbers return to normal. Oestrogen, therefore, has a neuroprotective role and research is exploring how the introduction of exogenous oestrogen may improve memory and reduce dementia risk.

Dementia is not normal brain aging but is due to a disease process. Dementia is an umbrella term which includes the many different types of neurological diseases whose symptoms include a gradual irreversible deterioration in brain function. Dementia is now termed neurocognitive disorder, and there are various types, such as Alzheimer's disease, vascular dementia, Lewy body dementia, Parkinson's dementia, HIV dementia, and many more.

Alzheimer's disease is the most common form of neurocognitive disorder, accounting for about seventy per cent of cases. There are many suggested causes of the disease, including lifestyle factors, genetics and hormonal ones. Alzheimer's disease is more prevalent in women than men, with women having two times greater lifetime risk of developing the disease. The risk for women increases after menopause, as they are older, and possibly due to hormonal causes.

As stated, there are brain-cell and brain-tissue-specific receptors that require oestrogen to operate. One of those areas of brain tissue where there are oestrogen receptors is also the site of Alzheimer's disease. The disease pathology is abnormal clusters of proteins that form plaques and tangles. Because of plaques and tangles, brain cells die and brain tissue shrinks. In laboratory studies oestrogen has been found to reduce plaque formation as well as reducing the number of tangles. Research also suggests that the genetic risk for Alzheimer's disease is more significant in women, as the particular genes have a greater influence on the development of disease pathology than they do in men.

Science bite: Oestrogen and Alzheimer's disease

The neuropathology of Alzheimer's disease (AD) involves plaques and tangles. Plaques are excessive beta amyloid deposits, which are caused by the faulty division of proteins and are toxic to brain cells. The tangles are neurofibrillary aggregates of hyperphosphorylated tau protein. It is suggested that oestrogens inhibit amyloid (amyloid β (Aβ) deposition), preventing the formation of plaques.

The established genetic risk for AD is ApoE4 (ε4). Apolipoproteins are proteins that bind lipids such as fat and cholesterol to make lipoproteins. In the central nervous system, ApoE4 is involved in the

---

transport of cholesterol to brain cells and is associated with amyloid deposition. Although it is still not clear exactly why, in women ApoE ε4 increases the probability of developing AD more than it does in men. Approximately forty to sixty-five per cent of adults with AD have at least one copy of ε4 allele – but not all do, so you can get AD without the genes. Those with two copies have an up to twenty times higher risk of developing AD, and the disease usually starts before age sixty-five and is termed early onset. It is not common and affects around five per cent of people with the disease. In older adults without AD fifteen per cent will have the ε4 allele variant and remain cognitively healthy. Lifestyle really counts.

The second most common form of dementia is vascular dementia due to cerebrovascular disease. Cerebrovascular disease is simply vascular disease of the brain in the same way that cardiovascular disease is vascular disease of the heart. The brain and heart share the same vascular system. The heart health section in Part 3 describes how menopause increases risks for cardiovascular disease; this section describes how women's heart health impacts their brain health.

Post-menopause, women are more at risk of cerebrovascular disease then men of the same age and experience more strokes and ischaemic brain changes. Women's health outcomes after a stroke are also worse than those for men. The health of our vascular system changes over our lifespan and with increasing age we are more sensitive to reduced blood flow (ischaemic change). A deficient supply of blood means less oxygen in the brain and causes brain cells to die. Before menopause women's risk of ischaemic changes is low, but after menopause our risk goes up.

There are several pathways via which menopause can increase risk for vascular dementia. The most obvious is the way in which oestrogen boosts vascular health by supporting the endothelium lining of blood vessels during adulthood, but then during the menopause transition there is less available oestrogen to carry out this protective function.

Another possible pathway is via the stress response. A reduction in oestrogen leads to increased activation of the stress response (sympathetic nervous system), which causes increased vascular tension (blood pressure). Increased blood pressure means it is more likely that the tiny blood vessels in the brain, which may be as fine as a strand of hair, are compromised and restrict the flow of oxygen and glucose to brain cells. The rate of hypertension (raised blood pressure) is lower in pre-menopausal women than in post-menopausal women, and sometimes even higher than in men of the same age.

Science bite: Oestrogen and vascular dementia

Lower levels of oestrogen lead to multiple risks for vascular health and stroke. In animals that have had their ovaries removed (to mimic menopause) it is not just the number of strokes that increases with loss of oestrogen but also that the damage caused by stroke increases. In contrast, female animals with oestrogen have fewer strokes but also have a more helpful immune response when they have a stroke – they do not have an excessive immune T-cell inflammatory response, which can worsen the damage.

Another suggested causal pathway linking oestrogen and dementia is that oestrogen increases the effective transport of fats in the bloodstream to the brain. The brain is nearly sixty per cent fat, and fatty acids are crucial for brain health and function. Essential fatty acids are so important that without them brain performance becomes impaired. Fatty acids are important for structure, but also for production of brain messengers and for the synthesis and function

---

of neurotransmitters. Oestrogen has been shown to influence the amount of essential fatty acids in the brain (docosahexaenoic acid, or DHA). Post-menopause, the transport diminishes, with the result that the brain may become under-fuelled. A simple remedy, though, is to boost your consumption of healthy omega-3 fatty acid foods so the available volume compensates for the poorer transport. Apart from the transport of fatty acids the neuroprotective benefits of oestrogen also include support of the vascular system itself. The brain requires plenty of oxygen and energy to function and these need to be transported via the vascular system, without which brain cells will die.

It is again more complicated. The same brain oestrogen receptors that control hypertension also regulate other vascular risk factors such as insulin, cholesterol, obesity and inflammation. All those risk factors are influenced by age and changing oestrogen levels, with women moving from low risk pre-menopause to high risk post-menopause. However, as already mentioned, menopause is a great time to improve your health and target risk factors that you can control through lifestyle, so that post-menopause you can be healthier than when you started!

To reduce your risk for vascular dementia it is necessary to improve your cardiovascular and cerebrovascular function. One key to that is to be a healthy weight. The second key is to improve your fitness levels through regular exercise, as this improves your entire cardiovascular system. Refer to Part 2 for further information on diabetes, weight and cholesterol and Part 3 for heart health.

Hormonal treatment for dementia

The idea that low oestrogen may be a risk factor for dementia has led researchers to explore the possibility that hormone therapy (HT) may change risk levels. Several population studies of groups of women already taking hormones suggest that the treatment favourably reduced dementia risk. Therefore, some researchers have suggested prescribing sex hormones as potential neuro-treatment for dementia. Researchers and pharmaceutical organisations have investigated oestrogen and progesterone, either in combination or individually. However, the results do not support using these hormones for this purpose. Prescribing hormones to women post-menopause to prevent normal age-related cognitive decline has produced inconsistent results, so no one is sure whether it works or not. The negative side effects associated with HT – increased risk for breast cancer, stroke and thromboembolic disease – are a major issue. Additionally, there is some research that suggests hormone treatment may possibly *increase* dementia risk.

For example, the MEDALZ Finnish study of more than 200,000 women examined the link between hormone treatment and Alzheimer's dementia and found no association. Another study reported higher risk for dementia in those taking hormones compared to those who were not. Furthermore, review of women's brain scans indicated that women who were taking hormone treatment had greater grey matter volume loss. In other brain structure examinations oestrogen therapy has been linked to brain shrinkage and increased white matter intensities that indicate vascular changes. Population studies like these are difficult to unpack because they are natural groups of women and there is no control of factors such as age, health and disease status that may also influence the results.

There have been several large-scale clinical trials, but the results remain equivocal even when those factors are controlled.

One of the findings was that the timing of HT introduction was important. An early study, the ELITE trial, compared treatment with early menopause (within six years) and compared it to women having treatment in late menopause (ten-plus years). The women were then split into groups based upon their health status on measures of metabolism, cholesterol, lipids and so forth and then given either progesterone or a placebo. Consistent with all other studies, those with the lowest health profile had the lower cognitive function whether they had HT or not. However, all those who received progesterone experienced some improvement in their general cognitive function and memory.

Another clinical trial comparing the introduction of oestrogen and progesterone with no treatment found that those receiving oestrogen had reduced Alzheimer's dementia pathology (amyloid burden) than those who did not receive oestrogen, and the benefits were particularly good for those who had been identified with the genetic risk. But there was no sign that their cognitive difficulties improved, just that disease pathology was lowered, so functionally it made no difference to women's lives.

Understanding the role of oestrogen may have significant implications for disease prevention and management. But at present no longer-term benefits of synthetic oestrogen therapy are clear. A prospective study that tracked women for twenty-two years found no improvement in cognitive function or reduced Alzheimer's dementia risk from HT. Cochrane reviews, held to be the highest level of investigation, do not recommend the use of hormones for neuroprotective purposes because there is no substantial evidence that the introduction of HT prevents dementia in women.

Oestrogen, menopause and the brain make up a new frontier in medical research, which is exciting. There is the promise that oestrogen may affect brain disorders in both men and women; however, there is still much to learn, and much of what you read now will be significantly expanded on in future. One aspect to consider in this conversation is age and study duration. Menopause occurs in midlife and women have decades of living after their last period, so we need to have more studies that last much longer than they currently do to separate the effects of age on the brain from menopause hormonal changes.

Until there is a cure or treatment for dementia we need to reduce our risks. Therefore, it is vital for women to develop a healthy lifestyle to optimise their brain health and cognitive performance. Thankfully there are many lifestyle strategies and options available, so we can develop a lifestyle pattern that suits our individual needs. Many of the healthy hormone strategies are outlined in Part 2 and expanded here to be specific to dementia risk. You can also read more about lifestyle and dementia risk reduction in my first book, *A Brain for Life*.

Self-care: Build your brain

- **Grow your brain with exercise.** Physical exercise is great for our bodies and our health, which is good for the brain. We also now know that exercise stimulates brain growth, and that a lack of physical exercise increases the risk of dementia by around fifteen per cent. Get moving and develop a regular exercise regime of at least three hours per week. Consider simply walking briskly if you are not a sporty person, but also think about taking up a recreational sport, joining a gym, learning to swim, cycling, and strength-based activities such as yoga, Pilates and weight training.
- **Fuel your brain.** Everything you eat affects your brain whether it is highly nutritious food that your brain requires to function properly or has low nutrition with high sugars, salts or fats. Diet impacts dementia risk. Consider eating the best fuel for your brain in the same

way you put the right fuel in your car. High protein, multiple vegetables and healthy oils are the best menu.

- **Sleep to learn.** When we are sleeping our brain is very busy. It is forming memories and consolidating what we know. Chronic sleep disturbance adversely affects memory, and long term it increases dementia risk. Lack of sleep stresses the brain and as a result several brain-determined body functions do not work so well. Aim for between seven and nine hours' sleep, develop a bedtime routine and care for your sleep hygiene.

- **Manage stress to protect your brain.** Manage your stress levels – there are no negative side effects to doing this. Reducing stress reactivity reduces blood pressure, reduces inflammation and reduces cortisol – three things that undermine brain health and increase dementia risk. Strategies to consider are to learn relaxation or mindfulness, being assertive and saying no, developing realistic expectations, improving problem solving, communicating and staying connected.

- **Boost memory.** To improve your memory, you can develop internal memory tricks or external compensation strategies. Internal strategies are things like repeating information, making up rhymes and mnemonics, making links and associations between new information and old, and chunking information into groups. External aids include things such as using calendars, writing to-do lists, keeping a diary, organising your personal affairs and keeping everything in a designated place (such as a bowl for keys by the front door).

- **Reduce brain burden.** Substance misuse through drinking too much alcohol, smoking cigarettes or using non-prescription drugs significantly reduces brain health. Ceasing smoking will reduce dementia risk by up to sixteen per cent, for example. Monitor your habits and make brain-positive choices.

- **Engage your brain.** The saying 'use it or lose it' is true. The brain loves challenges and stimulation to grow and adapt. Engage in interesting and stimulating hobbies and activities that build brain resilience.

Mood and mind

Mood swings are often a characteristic of female puberty and they are also reported by women going through the menopausal transition. The significant shifts in hormone levels at both ends of our reproductive life stage change how women feel and react. There is a pervasive general belief that women are moodier than men and the changing nature of the female mood is attributed to their female hormones. However, being emotionally reactive and receptive is not necessarily the same as being moody. Suffering from stress, mental health challenges or mental illness is not being moody either. The use of the word moody is not always helpful and can be disempowering. We *all* need to nurture our emotional wellbeing and mental health. The hormonal surges that we experience can impact our mood and mental wellbeing, making us vulnerable, so we need to take extra care of our minds.

Emotional response

Emotions, and emotional recognition, evolved for human survival. Mother Nature is not sloppy, and each emotion has a fundamental role in our health and wellbeing. Female hormones, through evolution, particularly support nurturing and make women emotionally attuned. The suggestion is that women's emotional strength ensures they are more attentive to the environment, empathic to children's needs and intuitive towards others' intentions, as this keeps them and their offspring safe. This capacity evolved because women have a physical strength disadvantage. While these attributes may be or have been valued in societies where attack, predators and tribal war may be or have been more likely, emotional sensitivity and responsiveness has increasingly been viewed as a weakness, and society generally appears less tolerant of emotional range, especially those that make us feel uncomfortable. In women their emotional difference to men is too often medicated, particularly during the transition.

Women's emotions are in a *natural* state of flux due to their hormonal changes, and for many during menses and menopause emotional sensitivity is heightened.

It is important that we celebrate the important role emotions have in our survival and wellbeing, and that we learn to accept them and allow them to pass. It is our emotional depth that makes us human. Rather than have emotions diagnosed as problems, perhaps we need to consider women's emotional reactivity as an essential sign of emotional health, and then work out ways to provide the best support and optimal management. It may or may not require pharmacological treatment.

Case study: Drama queen

My mother had an early menopause, but I was not quite ready to be told in my late thirties that I was peri-menopausal. It seemed as if I suddenly moved from a young to an 'old' woman. For someone who had not married until I was thirty-three, and after three pregnancies that resulted in no children, this came as a bit of a blow – OK, it was devastating. Some of my friends were still having children and I was on the way to hot flushes!

Hubby and I sat down and discussed the fact that we might not have a family in quite some detail, particularly as he is ten years my junior. We also discussed alternative options for having our family, but dismissed them for various reasons. Adoption was not an option due to our 'average' age.

From that point, we decided to see what happened – if we had children they would be welcomed, if not we would just be the greatest aunt and uncle we could be. That was the right approach, and no, he didn't leave for a younger model.

In my mid-forties the factory slowed and gradually stopped production – my periods, which were of the 'set the calendar' regularity, came, or didn't come, to their own schedule and I started the dreaded hot flushes. Oh, what joy they were!

My new-age, very loving husband was not always a help! Seeing what was happening, he would reach for the largest, whitest napkin and dab my face – just in case anyone around me had missed the waterfall from my hairline to my décolletage, hubby helped them see the phenomenon – woman turns into waterfall!

Otherwise, I was relatively lucky – my doctor and I agreed I would not take hormones unless the menopause symptoms stopped me from doing things I wanted and needed to do, such as going to work.

In a way, I was too busy for menopause to take over my life. When all is said and done, menstruation and menopause are forty or more years of your lifespan: far too long to allow them to be other than a natural event, not a big deal. I never allowed periods to rule my life, I certainly wasn't going to allow menopause to take control.

The week I turned fifty I started to bleed and three weeks later I was still bleeding, passing huge clots. I was booked for a D&C, but a few days before I was due in hospital, I stopped bleeding. Although the procedure went ahead, that was the end of menopause. No more periods, no more hot flushes, just tears.

Yes, that's right, tears. Menopause caused a huge change in my personality – I became a crier! 'Oh, look at the beautiful sunset,' tears in eyes; 'Isn't that a beautiful tribute?' (to someone I don't know), more tears; 'I'm so happy!' Then why am I crying? Yes, the manufacturers of tissues have benefited greatly from my change of life.

Specific areas of the brain (hippocampus, hypothalamus and amygdala) influenced by sex hormones impact upon a woman's mood, self-esteem and how she connects to others. Changes in hormones may also change behaviour, emotional regulation and how a woman feels and responds to stress. While some subtle changes in mood are experienced by many women during the transition, for a minority menopause is a real time of risk for poor mental health and diminished quality of life.

There are several different ways in which the menopausal transition may change a woman's normal emotional equilibrium and mental health. The most obvious pathway is that the loss of oestrogen and progesterone directly changes mood. The next likely cause is that the physical symptoms of menopause such as disturbed sleep, loss of libido, and hot sweats drain a woman's resilience and leave her more vulnerable to stress and overwhelm her ability to cope. It can become a vicious cycle as symptoms increase stress which worsens symptoms. The other link is that the changes in oestrogen and progesterone impact upon other hormones and neurotransmitters, some of which support normal mood along with feelings of attachment and joy. Sometimes this is worsened by how we think about and judge our ability to cope, and our responses may contribute to a negative spiral of mood changes, self-criticism, shame and loss of self-esteem. Other times it may be the responses of partners and others that are unhelpful and it is the quality of our relationships that influence our mental wellbeing.

We need a circuit breaker. Self-understanding and self-compassion. A mindful menopause transition will help us bloom. There are many things that women can do to protect themselves and feel better. In fact, menopause is an opportunity to do things differently, better manage stress, think more positively, and we may be even feel better than ever before. So, let's understand our hormones, mood and stress with an open mind and non-judgemental heart – in other words let's be kind to ourselves.

Case study: Hot then blue

I was having a terrible time with menopause. For three months I would have hot flushes then no more. But I would then have months of depression. Then hot flushes again and then depression again.

I asked if my depression was menopausal and my doctor said no. I lasted two years and then saw a psychologist. I was telling her about my depression and she asked where I was in menopause. I immediately said, 'I knew it.' Her question had just confirmed my suspicion. She sent me back to my doctor to investigate hormone treatment and we started to work on my depression. Therapy really helped as I was able to look at my thinking patterns and make some goals. Prioritising my health, taking hormones and kick-starting my exercise again got me through.

Science bite: Stress hormones

The stress response is due to activation of the hypothalamic–pituitary–adrenal (HPA) system: the hypothalamus, pituitary gland and adrenal gland respectively. This system is vital for normal body homeostasis as it regulates the cardiovascular, immune and metabolic systems. When we are exposed to stress the hypothalamus releases corticotropin-releasing hormone (CRH), which in turn triggers the pituitary to release adrenocorticotropic hormone (ACTH), which then sends a message to the adrenal gland to produce cortisol (glucocorticoids) and adrenaline. Cortisol and adrenaline then activate several other physiological systems in order to enhance our ability to adapt, cope and survive. This is an important feedback–feedforward loop so the system can be turned up or down depending upon need. Knowledge is limited, however it appears that oestrogen receptors impact the HPA axis. Additionally, as it is a steroid hormone, oestrogen influences other hormones. For example, a decrease in oestrogen is linked to an increase in cortisol and adrenaline. An oestrogen decrease is also linked to a decrease in endorphins, oxytocin and serotonin (all of which, when present in adequate amounts, contribute to us feeling positive).

Case study: Really bad place

I am in menopause and I hate it. I have cotton wool in my head. I do really worry about dementia all the time, especially as my mother had dementia. Both my sister and I worry about it as our memories are not what they used to be. I just can't remember things at work like I used to. Everything takes so long as I do remember eventually, but I am essentially all over the shop at work, not on an even keel at all.

*I can deal with the hot flushes as they come and pass.
I don't like the anxiety as it feels like a weight, or tightness
around my shoulders and neck. I do not like that feeling of
uneasiness and constantly not being relaxed. I just feel like
things are not right all the time.*

*A few weeks ago, I had a feeling of dread. I had not
been there before as I usually see beauty in a drop of water.
But this time I was in a really bad place for a week. At that
point I did not want to talk to anybody as I was ashamed of
how low I felt – I thought what is the point being here and
that terrified me. It was so unlike me. Later my partner was
quite shocked by how bad I was. I went to my doctor and
blood tests revealed that my hormones had suddenly really
dropped down.*

Stress and menopause

Stress impacts female hormones and female hormones impact stress. Stress worsens menopause, menopause may worsen stress, and menopause may cause the stress. Let's face it, symptoms like hot flushes, night sweats, migraines, vaginal dryness, weight gain and loss of libido are not easy to cope with!

Stress impacts our entire body, including hormone production and regulation. When our inner and outer lives are going smoothly we usually feel calm and comfortable, and perhaps content. Ideally this is how we feel most of the time. When we are not stressed our brain–body–mind function is kept at a healthy balanced level of wellbeing, managed by the parasympathetic nervous system (just think 'p' for peaceful). When life throws us a curve ball, be it physical, like being in pain, tired or sick, or when it is psychological due to loss, our thoughts and responses, or due to unmanageable demands on us or problems, our brain–body–mind switches from the calm operating system to the stress system, termed the

149

sympathetic nervous system (think 's' for stress). Activation of the stress system helps us to survive and cope and is often referred to as the fight or flight response (and there is freeze response too).

No matter what is causing the stress response to be activated, the physiological effects are ultimately the same. Inside the brain, messengers trigger the release of adrenaline and cortisol, and these then communicate with other body systems, such as the cardiovascular, immune, gastrointestinal and metabolic systems. They all help us get into survival mode, so we can deal with whatever is making us stressed. Activation of the stress response boosts our physical, mental and emotional functioning so we can fix the challenge/s we are facing. In most cases we can ultimately find a solution or resolution: we may need to recruit support from others, or problem solve what is making us stressed, use resources, or we may simply adapt and get used to it. Our stress levels go down and ideally we return to the calm, peaceful operating system.

A little activation of the stress response is positive and beneficial as it boosts our responses. However, when the stress response is chronically on and unremitting, there are high amounts of circulating cortisol and adrenaline in our system and the stress response becomes a major health burden.

What we consider stressful and how we respond to stress varies considerably from person to person and the differences are due to factors such as age, socioeconomic status, culture, religion, genetics and our sex hormones. Sometimes, medication can trigger the stress response and is impossible to control, so the reaction to the physiological arousal is important because we can increase or decrease the stress response.

Although the stress pathway is always the same, it is often divided into either psychological *or* physiological. This is not necessarily helpful, nor accurate as new research proves. The combined field of study which examines stress, neurology and hormones is called psycho-neuro-endocrinology and explores the interplay between mind, brain and body. An extreme example of how these three factors are linked is the way in which severe stress in women during their reproductive years lowers their fertility. While we now understand this, it took some time to discover the relationship between stress and our female hormones because the early stress-biology models included only male rodents. This situation has changed with the stipulation that female animals must be included in such studies. The results confirm that mental health and mood are, like everything in this book, related to multiple factors, including sex hormones and hormonal changes.

Case study: Fertility and stress do not mix well

The year I turned twenty-four everything changed. That was the year I had a (benign) brain tumour removed and was also diagnosed with premature ovarian failure, otherwise known as premature menopause.

The brain surgery, while very traumatic prior to diagnosis, with constant headaches, double vision and doctors telling me I was 'just stressed', and then the intensity of surgery, was over with after a few short months. On the other hand, the reality of being told that my ovaries had shut down for some unknown reason, and to just use a donor egg, was a much harder situation to handle and accept. Add to that the challenge of finding donors in Australia with our laws.

Putting aside my desire for a family for a moment, it was almost as hard emotionally facing doctors telling me my body was behaving like that of a fifty-year-old. And bless the surgeons for saving my life, but it wasn't the easiest thing to hear – 'It's fine! Just use a donor egg. Oh, and get counselling because you will need that.' Heavens, if only I could tell my twenty-four-year-old self how to get through that difficult time from where I am today at (almost) forty-one.

Earlier in the year of my tumour I was working hard in a stressful tech job in Sweden. I was flying in/out of Stockholm for an intense contract. Meanwhile I came off the pill after approximately a year. I don't recall if my periods returned prior to the headaches and intensity of that timeframe. I do recall the hot flushes started around then, as did the vaginal dryness. Oh, how I hated putting on a jumper for five minutes and then having to take it off five minutes later. Other people just didn't seem to understand. Especially people my age. Let alone receiving a prescription for HRT and being told you will get ovarian cancer if you don't take it. Then reading elsewhere that if you do take it, you are more likely to get breast cancer.

In hindsight it doesn't surprise me that I wanted to find the root cause. I tried alternative methods from here to the sun. I detoxed and saw a naturopath for eight months. I had my counselling/psychotherapy. I learned Reiki. I tried Gestalt therapy. I had craniosacral therapy. Later, I had countless acupuncture sessions to see if my ovaries would kick-start. No matter what, I didn't have the right man in my life and my motto became: No egg, no sperm, too hard. I know there are other women who wouldn't let that stop them but frankly while I really wanted children desperately I couldn't fathom choosing to be a single mum. I didn't want that for myself or for any child of mine.

It took me quite a number of years to meet the man I wanted to share my life with, and for him it took quite some time to come around to the idea of an egg donor. And fair enough. I'd had many years to come to terms with it.

My egg donor baby is so precious and loved and she is such a blessing in our life. I did have ongoing acupuncture during my IVF treatment and was told that the lining of my uterus was very good for the transfer, which it was

*clearly very successful. We are planning to repeat the IVF
experience in the near future with our frozen embryos and
hope that the second takes as easily as the first.*

*I really question how much the stress I experienced
during that year had a part to play in my ovaries switching
off. I can't help but think how smart nature is and how
fertility and stress do not mix well.*

Stress, as we have already seen, causes a reduction of progesterone
and oestrogen, and both of these female hormones influence mood.
Oestrogen is described as 'nature's psycho-protectant' because of
its de-stress effect. In men under stress, testosterone that enters
the brain is naturally converted to oestrogen, which lowers their
stress. Similarly, when people are given oestrogen replacement they
experience lower stress too. Progesterone too has a sedative, relaxing
and anti-anxiety effect, which also reduces stress responding.

The interwoven complexity continues. Serotonin is important
for normal mood. Stress reduces serotonin, and oestrogen influences
how much serotonin we have. Oestrogen affects serotonin levels via
different pathways so when oestrogen goes down during menopause
serotonin goes down too. When stress goes up oestrogen,
progesterone and serotonin go down. Now enter menopause. In
peri-menopause, oestrogen, progesterone and serotonin fluctuate
and menopause starts, and when oestrogen and progesterone go
down, serotonin dips and stress goes up. Taken together, no wonder
the fluctuations and ultimate reduction of these hormones during
the menopausal transition can leave some women feeling stressed,
anxious or sad, or that their mood goes up and down like a roller
coaster. It is believed that it is the fluctuations that cause the most
detrimental impact – a slow reduction is less problematic.

Added to this are the knock-on effects to other hormones. The
increased production of cortisol during stress means that there
are fewer resources available to make other vital hormones for a

healthy body and mind, along with decreased immune function and increased inflammation. A group of hormones that particularly suffer are those associated with positive mood. These are the four feel-good hormones of blissful endorphins, pleasurable dopamine, connection oxytocin and normal mood serotonin. Going in the opposite direction are the negative consequences of increased adrenaline, which impairs sleep, which increases fatigue, which contributes to brain fog, and all of this reduces the body's ability to rest and restore. Not surprisingly this exacerbates your stress load and the whole negative cycle starts again.

For some women symptoms, and their responses to them, and possibly a lack of compassionate support, can make menopause stressful. A six-year study published in the journal *Menopause* found that stress and anxiety preceded hot flushes and that higher stress levels were related to increased flushes – both in frequency and intensity. Stress levels are also related to night sweats. The interpretation is that women who worry suffer more. It can also become cyclical, whereby the prospect of flushes occurring causes stress and anxiety which leads to them occurring.

Case study: Hard road

I have never taken the easy road in anything in my seventy-three years; it now makes me laugh when I look back on my life. My journey into menopause began when I was about to marry again when I was forty-seven.

The first 'hot flush' hit me so hard. It was an explosive ten minutes or so – I was in bed at the time, luckily, as at the end of the hot flush, my heart was racing, I was giddy and felt completely drained and my nightie was saturated as were my sheets.

I had not even prepared my mind for menopause. I was young and happy, a mother of two adult daughters and had no indication that this new phase of my life named 'menopause' had struck me. My periods had always been erratic, I was underweight, and had been all my life. My periods had not begun until after I turned sixteen.

I thought I might be 'coming down with something' and put it out of my mind. I was planning a wedding after all. As the weeks went by these episodes continued until they became so bad they consumed me. Each episode lasted at least ten minutes and always the hot flush was like the first one and left me in the same state.

The day my condition dawned on me was at a time when I was having the hot flushes in more frequent intervals, even as close as twenty minutes apart. I made an appointment to see my local doctor, he confirmed my fear it was the dreaded 'menopause'.

The doctor wrote out a prescription for hormone replacement tablets, which relieved the symptoms after a month or so. I returned to normal and went on with my plan to marry.

That did not go well. Years passed, and I rebuilt my life, still taking the hormone replacement tablets and now antidepressants until one day when I was sixty my doctor changed my antidepressants to Avanza as he said they were not addictive and that Xanax were, within months while I was taking the Avanza I was really relaxed and happy.

Unfortunately, my weight increased from fifty-four kilos to eighty-three kilos, so the doctor changed my antidepressants once more, which I took from then on. I was still taking the hormone replacement, the doctor took me off these and the hot flushes began again, so I begged him to write me a prescription; he did.

My life went on happily this way until I was sixty-two and I began to bleed from my vagina, the doctor took me off the hormone replacement tablets altogether. I did have a few hot flushes from time to time until I was seventy, although nothing like before.

I was still taking the antidepressants as I was having panic attacks and since I had stopped the hormone replacement my panic attacks had increased. I had put the increase of panic attacks down in part to my partner of twenty years being terminally ill.

After my partner's death last year, I forgot to get a prescription for the antidepressants as I was grieving and so I stopped taking them. Surprisingly, I have not had a panic attack or hot flush since.

I should add that I have never had any other symptoms other than the hot flushes. My blood pressure is perfect, and I do not take any tablets at all now, not even a Panadol.

In women the part of the brain that responds to stress and panic (locus coeruleus) is larger. This part of the brain is responsible for the production of noradrenaline and may explain why women have higher levels of cortisol than men in response to stress. Animal studies also suggest that males and females react differently to stress. Specifically, males are reportedly more likely to engage in 'fight or flight' behaviour while females are more likely to 'tend or befriend'. This research is both novel and controversial. The theoretical explanation is that females have more oxytocin (because of oestrogen), so they act in a calm protective way and/or seek help, in particular to protect their young. In contrast, males have more testosterone so are thought to respond in a more active 'defensive/aggressive' manner. Functional imaging studies where stress exposure is manipulated confirm differences in decision-making processes, learning and feedback as brain activation patterns differ between the brains of women and men.

It is one thing to manipulate stress responding in a study and another thing entirely in real life. However, and unfortunately, there are real-life opportunities to study differences in stress responses. In 2016, an Australian study was published examining the difference between men's and women's responses to the tragic 2009 Black Saturday bushfires in Victoria. Overall, men tended to underestimate or play down the risk and had a preference to stay and defend their property, while women were more likely to listen to and act on advice and leave. A survey of bushfire civilian deaths in Australia indicates that men are almost three times more likely to die than women. This suggests that in some situations, like bushfires, the best response for survival is to listen and leave. In other situations, it may be appropriate to fight and defend. As stated at the beginning of this book, the differences between men and women, which are few, should be viewed as complementary strengths.

These differences in behaviour have only been evident in response to acute stress events or crisis situations and appear to disappear in non-crises. The longer-term consequences of chronic high stress are the same for both men and women – it reduces physical health and mental wellbeing and is a significant risk factor for depression and mental illness. Which means we all need to reduce our exposure to grinding stress and manage stress as it arises, so our mental health does not deteriorate. Furthermore, stress does not equate with mental illness per se, so there is no need for psychotropic medication, but rather for acceptance of emotional range, stress management and perhaps hormone management.

Mental health

The hormone dance of peri-menopause and menopause can lead to increased risk for mental illness such as depression. Women are two and a half times more likely to present with major depression than men. Some differences, especially in symptoms, are now linked to changes in hormone levels. During peri-menopause and in the five to six years after a woman's last period in post-menopause, depression risk is especially high.

Depression is associated with lower levels and less effective use of serotonin in the brain. Oestrogen influences serotonin receptors. Therefore, it follows that women are at risk of depression when their oestrogen levels are low – early pregnancy, post-partum and during the menopause transition, or when oestrogen is low compared to progesterone, which is the luteal phase of the menstrual cycle.

Mental health status prior to the onset of menopause, and probably peri-menopause too, is an important factor. Those women with prior mental health challenges and/or a history of mental illness have a higher risk of developing difficulties during the transition. The nature of menopause onset also influences risk of mental illness. Women going through natural menopause have lower risk of depression and anxiety compared to those who undergo medical menopause. Whilst the length of time to complete the menopause transition is not a significant factor influencing depression risk, the number and severity of menopausal symptoms is.

The evidence about menopause and depression risk is very recent. In the past women's vulnerability and menopausal depression may have been largely ignored or treated inappropriately as the association between menopause and mental health was only officially recognised last decade. The American College of Obstetricians and Gynecologists only stated in 2009 that *the constant change of hormone levels during this time can have a troubling effect on emotions ... leaving some women to feel irritable and even depressed*. However, many mental health professionals have still not caught up with this message. In February 2017, a psychological society article stated that *sex-based risks to mental health have been overlooked*, indicating that the lack of understanding of how sex hormones impact mental health continues.

Case study: Sleepless

I think menopause unto itself is manageable, although unpleasant. I think the story people don't think of is how it impacts on other aspects of health. We treat menopause as an issue, but it is its effects that can be the problem.

I was maybe fifty-two when I thought I was in peri-menopause because I was waking at night in hot sweats. I had a period maybe eight months ago, and I don't think I'll have another one – but I've said that before. But I am going to be fifty-five next month and it's just an intuition thing, I think they're gone.

At the beginning I did want to do something about the hot flushes because lack of sleep became an issue. And it still is an issue. I have been sick for six weeks with pneumonia and it's taking so long to get well because of lack of sleep. It just steals my ability to restore myself.

I have got a bit of anxiety and when I wake in the middle of the night with a hot flush it's the anxiety that keeps me awake if I am in an anxious period of life. My anxiety is keeping me up so I can't get enough sleep. My anxiety is more prevalent now, but I am not sure if it is strictly based on my hormones or life circumstances too – such as looking for work at age fifty-five, moving to a new house, and my husband losing his job.

I go and see a psychologist once a month and CBT has been the best thing for my anxiety. At least I can function, and I can manage. The only thing I have not done is take medication for anxiety, but I came really close when I got sick.

Women are prescribed more mood medications than men, and especially when women are aged between thirty-five and sixty-four, which coincides with peri-menopause and menopause.

According to American data approximately one in four women take a psychiatric medication, compared with one in seven men. Similarly, a study reviewing the rates of hospitalisation for psychotic disorders between men and women found the same age effect. Examination of the rates of acute hospital admissions over three years found that women older than fifty-five had higher proportions of hospitalisation and were prescribed higher doses of psychotropic medications than men of the same age.

In other cases, women are prescribed medication when they are simply responding naturally to unnatural demands – too much work, poverty or inability to provide for their children, too little support from partners, lack of social contact, or lifestyle factors like poor diet, limited exercise or time outside in the sunshine. Their warning system – emotions – is saying that something is not right. Appropriately addressing the issue/s is necessary. Some issues can be addressed at an individual level; however, issues like violence against women, poverty of single mothers, parental leave and wage equity need to be addressed at a societal level. Prior to prescribing psychiatric medication it is important to consider women's normal hormonal changes, healthy emotional reactions, lifestyle, environment and socioeconomic and political factors. Medications may improve mental health for many women with mental illnesses but should be a sensible medical decision, not one based upon a limited view of emotional responding, marketing by pharmaceutical companies, or a perception that there are no other options. Many lifestyle and mindstyle changes are effective interventions. For example, recent studies internationally and within Australia demonstrate that the introduction of a highly nutritious diet will reduce depression. Additionally, for many people with depression, cognitive behaviour therapy which improves mindstyle is more effective than medication.

Medication no doubt improves and saves lives. However, examination of prescriptions indicates that psychiatric medications are increasingly being prescribed by non-psychiatrists who may not understand the associations between stress, sex hormones and mental health, and thereby may over-prescribe psychiatric medication when other treatments could be utilised, and which have less severe side effects.

In recent years there have been major health statements made by psychiatrists warning doctors not to just prescribe mood drugs but to think about menopause management too. Hormone treatment during the transition may make a big difference to a woman's mental health and has lower-level side effects than psychiatric medications. Combining antidepressant treatment for women with depression during menopause and hormone treatment is helpful and the amounts prescribed of both medications may be less for the same impact. However, this type of combined treatment is not actively pursued, largely due to ignorance. There are also non-pharmacological options too. For example, education and reassurance. If anxiety starts or increases it does not mean that there is an anxiety disorder per se that needs medicating. Rather, women will benefit from understanding the anxiety response, that their anxiety levels will naturally vary, and that this variation is normal. Understanding that the heightened feelings of emotion and anxiety are physiological and will pass can make a big impact upon a woman's coping and resilience. The assurance that you are not going mad and that your symptoms are due to chemical changes can have a profound benefit. Anxiety management strategies and cognitive behaviour therapy, as well as a mental health enhancing lifestyle, may be more helpful and effective than medication. From my own experience of medical menopause, stopping coffee, keeping positive, soothing self-talk and prioritising sleep got me through attacks of physiological panic linked to medication side effects.

Case study: Mood magnification

I had a client who had been involved in a horrific single-vehicle accident. The vehicle she was in had slid on loose gravel, left the road and rolled six times before colliding with a tree. She had several soft-tissue injuries and a neck injury but no fractures or organ trauma. She also had no memory of the accident, which for her was a good thing. After about twelve months all her injuries had settled down, although she was left with constant chronic pain in her neck and shoulder.

I saw her three years after the accident. She still had ongoing pain and a large number of what could be termed mood symptoms including sadness, crying, feeling depressed, worry, fear and a sense of isolation. She had also gained weight, lost interest in sex, and had disturbed sleep. All these can indicate a psychological illness, and she had been diagnosed with adjustment disorder.

Given her age I asked her where she was in the menopausal transition. She was surprised. However, she realised she was possibly in peri-menopause at the time of her accident but was experiencing full menopausal symptoms now. Minutes after this conversation she had a hot flush in my office and laughed. We stopped, and she flapped and fanned herself, and had a cool wet towel. When she felt 'back to normal' we proceeded.

We started to unpack what was happening for her not just in terms of the accident but also in terms of her life and hormonal journey. One thing became immediately apparent: no treating or specialist reviewing doctor had asked her about her menopause status.

The other significant factor was that she was experiencing an overwhelming number of symptoms attributable to menopause that were not being treated. The symptoms were all presumed to be due to the accident, or her response to it, when in fact they could also be due to menopause. Either way they could be treated.

Importantly, she reported that her response to her situation was not characteristic of her. She felt an alien within herself. She could not explain why her emotional response was so severe, especially given she had no memory of the accident. She said that she 'should be better', and added, 'Depression – I think I've got under control – good days and bad days – but my anxiety is off the charts.'

I asked how she was managing her symptoms and she said she was using natural remedies that were not working.

I explained how our hormones oestrogen and progesterone impact our mood, and that during menopause anxiety and depression were significant issues for some women. I suggested her depression and anxiety may in part be due to her menopausal status AND the accident. I also suggested that by treating her hormones we could reduce some of the symptoms she was experiencing and then focus on what was remaining – adjusting to the accident, pain and anxiety.

As a result, she went back to her treating doctor. We ended up having a round-table discussion and she went on hormone replacement. Several issues immediately improved, and she also received psychological therapy for her anxiety and developed very effective stress-management strategies including a health-boosting menopause lifestyle.

Menopause can make a difficult time harder to manage if neglected and may worsen a situation that is already tricky. It may drain energy and deplete internal resources and make it very hard to manage other life stresses. The best tactic to manage mental wellbeing is therefore to care for it every day and prevent issues becoming insurmountable. But women often ignore their own health as they are busy caring for others. Instead think about prioritising your mental wellbeing with the same care and regularity you care for your teeth – a few minutes once or twice a day. Check in with yourself daily, review your stress levels, and reduce or manage unwanted stress.

What worked in the past may need to be enhanced and augmented as the menopausal transition is naturally reducing your reserves with or without any stressors being present in your life. The other essential tip is to be very mindful of how high your acute short-stress response is so that it does not tip over into a chronic pattern of stress responding and a potential mental health issue.

Because hormones are fluctuating and may be affecting your thinking it may also be helpful to perhaps withhold making major life decisions until a calm balance is reached. Having heightened emotional responding and being under stress inhibits thinking and problem-solving ability to make the best choice. Although functional studies suggest that brain activation changes during hormonal fluctuations to assist women to think, make decisions and monitor emotions, the stress response has the opposite effects. I suggest where possible that women wait until they are in their best place to make decisions to meet their longer-term goals.

The ultimate message from this section is to actively manage stress and proactively treat and manage mental health issues such as depression and anxiety, which increase during the transition. We must also appreciate that no matter how bad the transition feels it will pass and we will get through. But it is up to us to help ourselves as best we can with what will be most helpful.

Self-care: Nurture mental wellbeing

- **Get control.** Menopause is a natural process but that does not mean you do not need help to get through. Do not let it overwhelm you: be proactive. Get help to manage your symptoms. Talk to registered health professionals who understand menopause and mood, so you can establish the best treatment regime for your individual needs. Review your plan regularly as things will change.
- **Keep a circle of friends.** Identify the positive, energising and supportive friends in your life. Include your partner in this circle too. Reach out to them and stay actively connected on a regular basis. Share the menopausal journey with others to increase understanding and kind compassion in your life – and laugh together too.
- **Learn to say no.** The menopause transition can change how you feel and sap your energy. Start saying no to things which are not in your best interests or take too much of your precious resources. Stop compulsive caring for others and direct your precious caring energy towards those that matter, including yourself. Learn to start nurturing your own wellbeing as a priority without feeling guilty afterwards. You are worth your own care.
- **Eat positive mood foods.** A healthy diet is good for your mental health. Certain foods have higher benefits. A good example is those that contain tryptophan – chicken and turkey, spinach, pumpkin and sesame seeds, eggs and tuna – as this supports serotonin production. B3 and B6 vitamins and magnesium are also essential.
- **Increase your antioxidants.** Help your body reduce oxidative stress and inflammation by eating antioxidant-rich and anti-inflammatory foods such as the blues and reds – think blueberries, cranberries, beetroot and turmeric.

- **Reduce stimulants and substances.** Support your body's ability to keep control over the stress response by cutting down on stimulants such as caffeine, chocolate, sugar and alcohol, which get your heart and body racing.
- **Sleep well.** Sleep is an important factor in hormone function and mental health. There are links between oestrogen, sleep and depression rates in peri-and post-menopausal women. See Part 2 for more on sleep.
- **Boost your gut health.** The health of our gut bacteria influences levels of serotonin and the stress response. A healthy gut improves mood and reduces stress and anxiety. Eat probiotics like yoghurt with live bacteria cultures to naturally improve your mood.
- **Take your time.** Stop having meals on the run and juggling everything at once. Do one thing at a time. Book regular holidays – a 'staycation' at home or an away holiday. Or just simply do something different and change the routine. Take time out for yourself away from family demands – even if it means sitting in the car for an hour alone – or you could sing, listen to music or even nap. Schedule in pyjama days – when you do the minimum and just simply rest. You will be less emotional and anxious, and become calmer and have a clearer, less foggy brain.
- **Find the joys.** Identify the things that make you feel positive, optimistic, happy etc. It could include catching up with friends or family, a bubble bath, pizza and a glass of red, movies, reading, gardening, music, walking in nature, being by the sea, watching comedy, and much more. Make a list of your joy-giving things – perhaps five options – and try to engage in at least one each week. We experience joyful events so that we learn to repeat them!

- **Exercise wisely.** Regular, gentle exercise is essential, but not excessive exercise. Consider reducing excessive high-intensity exercise as this can burn through important adrenal supplies necessary to convert to oestrogen. Think about a mixed program of resistance and aerobic training, which benefits heart, bones and muscles, along with yoga or stretching for limbs and ligaments. They all improve brain and mind.

- **Learn how to relax.** With such busy fast-paced lives many find it difficult to simply pause. Focusing on having a calm steady breath is important – slowly inhale, pause and exhale slowly and work up to a count of four for each. Become a daydreamer and simply *be*, or learn more formal techniques such as progressive muscle or guided imagery meditation.

- **Self-soothe.** Develop a gentle, supportive inner voice that helps calm and soothe you, reassures you that you are doing okay and you are safe, believes in your ability to manage whatever life throws at you, and reminds you to keep perspective and focus on what is important to you.

- **Get skilled up.** Learn stress management, mindfulness or problem-solving strategies – or other things that may reduce stress like improving your financial literacy. You could also complete a cognitive behavioural therapy program for anxiety and depression or an acceptance commitment therapy course with a registered psychologist. It's as good as medication but without the negative side effects.

Science bite: Four positives

Although many hormones and neurotransmitters are involved in mood, there are four easily identifiable ones that we rely upon to feel pleasure, and which we can actively influence.

Dopamine gives us a crucial reward of pleasure – it makes us feel good. It also motivates us because it feels good. Find the things that give you joy, pleasure and a sense of reward. Celebrate your achievements, set and meet goals, engage in enjoyable activities and hobbies like music, dancing, favourite foods, sexual pleasure, and spending time with loved ones.

Serotonin supports normal mood and social behaviour. Simple exposure to sunlight increases serotonin so we are energised and have normal mood. Serotonin also flows when we have meaning and purpose or feel significant and vital, so find activities that give a sense of purpose and achievement. If you don't have any current ones, investigate options or simply think of past ones as the brain response is the same, past and present.

Oxytocin is what builds trust, connection to others, intimacy and healthy relationship bonds. Spend time with people you love, remind yourself how loved you are and relish emotional security. Smile at people and they will smile back – it helps. Boost oxytocin further by having hugs and cuddles for at least ten seconds, or have a massage, facial or other form of caring physical contact.

Endorphins trigger the release of positive feelings and have an analgesic effect. They are released in response to pain and stress to help alleviate anxiety and depression. Exercise is a fantastic way to release endorphins, as are high-thrill activities like sky-diving, but laughing also works. Watch a comedy, laugh and joke and spend time with funny people who laugh – it is contagious.

Attitude

Our mental attitude has a big impact on our emotional experience and mental wellbeing. Thoughts determine how we feel and they change our brain and body. Every thought becomes manifest in our body. For example, studies show increased antibody response after the flu vaccine in people with an optimistic outlook compared to those with a pessimistic view. A positive attitude immediately improves your physical health and mental wellbeing.

Now consider how much the thoughts and beliefs that you carry around all the time may influence your emotions and body. Worrying or pessimistic thoughts, fear and negative judgements disrupt our equilibrium with feelings of concern and anxiety and turn on stress. Optimistic, hopeful and positive thoughts bring a feeling of contentment and calmness. Our thoughts are so incredibly powerful that we can easily forget we have control over them and not the other way around.

Menopause is such a significant passage in life that we need to check our thoughts and attitudes regarding it, and aging more generally, as some thoughts may not be helpful. Ideally, we need to develop and maintain a positive frame of mind. This is because a negative frame of mind has a profoundly negative influence on our menopause experience. Attitude, including anticipation of a negative experience, makes a difference to how things are perceived in real time. Women who expect significant issues during menopause usually experience significant issues – it becomes self-fulfilling. Studies indicate that attitude – or mindstyle – is directly related to the number and severity of menopause symptoms, along with psycho-social and lifestyle factors.

A population study that tracked women for five years while going through the transition indicated that a fraction over half had positive attitudes towards menopause and one quarter had a negative attitude; the remainder were neutral. Clearly, most women are keeping a balanced if not positive view, which is wonderful given the history of menopause in medicine.

Dr Robert Wilson wrote a book called *Feminine Forever*, published in 1966, and he described menopause as a 'crippling disease' and a 'natural plague', and stated that women in post-menopause were 'crippled castrates'. This book received a lot of coverage, with the basic idea being that menopausal women were no longer sexually attractive or able to reproduce and were, therefore, impaired. Coinciding with his book was the entry of hormone therapy pills into the market. Dr Wilson had links to the pharmaceutical industry and specifically to hormone treatment, so his critical campaign was self-serving. Advertisers took up his arguments and played on women's vulnerability and fear of becoming unattractive and old. One particularly loathsome advertisement reportedly stated, 'she is concerned about losing her youth … and maybe about losing her husband.' The ubiquitous message to women in menopause and midlife was make yourself young or risk becoming sexually unattractive, old and alone.

With medical messages, cynical marketing campaigns and pejorative language about women in midlife, it is little wonder that many women dread menopause. Acceptance of the transition is a crucial step. You can't fight it. Like increasing age, it is a natural process and occurs regardless of what you do. We also get through it, with the Massachusetts Women's Health Study of more than 2500 women finding that post-menopause, most women felt relieved, or neutral as it was never an issue to start with.

Channel your precious energy into how to best manage the process for yourself rather than into dread or concern. I also suggest taking one more step and not only accepting the menopause transition but embracing it as an opportunity to take the time to improve your physical and mental wellbeing. Decide that menopause is a step forwards in your life, acknowledge and accept any difficulties and manage them as necessary, but think of the positives – it will end, for one. You may need some help and reminders to develop a more self-caring view but make it work, as the wellbeing benefits are priceless.

Case study: Mother's attitude

My first exposure to menopause, like many women, was listening to my mother's ongoing battle with it. From all accounts it was a horrible experience that caused her to put on weight and experience terrible night sweats. She learned quickly that to save herself from changing the sheets every night she would need to sleep on layers of towels.

It was so bad she invested in air-conditioning throughout the house. She was constantly wringing with sweat at the slightest movement. It was so bad, she would need a fan in the bathroom pointed directly at her like a jet engine just to apply her make-up, only to have it melt off her face as the day progressed.

In the end she refused to go anywhere without air-conditioning. That meant no outdoor cafes or restaurants, no sunset strolls or quick walks up to the shops to get milk. And I'm not just talking summer. We are talking about three hundred and sixty-five days, 24/7. It drove my mother nuts.

The whole family watched this happen not quite understanding where our outgoing and independent mother had gone. The merits of any outing were measured against her discomfort. And visiting her meant taking a cardigan to protect ourselves from her frosty air-conditioning.

I knew these symptoms faded over time but not for our mother. She is now eighty-one and still maintains a strict set of guidelines about body heat to sweat ratio for all activities and outings. I did try to point out that she should be well through menopause by now. She looked quite startled at the idea and maintains she is still going through it.

There are several important things that might be helpful with developing a positive accepting attitude and keeping menopause in perspective for young women and those already experiencing menopause. Menopause indicates health. Not going through menopause means you have been infertile and/or had serious health problems. No one misses out – all those born biologically female will go through menopause. Being judgmental makes things worse. There are no confirmed negative longer-term consequences of menopause if optimal health and wellbeing are maintained. Menopause cannot be controlled but we can manage and alleviate symptoms. The transition takes time and it can't be made to pass any faster. But it will pass.

Many wonderful things can happen with menopause. The realisation that the crazy cycling of hormones is over means women have clarity of mind and self-possession again – no more brain fog, no more being hijacked by hormones. Post-fertility affords many women the freedom to pursue their own goals and enjoy their sexuality without issues of contraception and pregnancy or having to take contraceptive hormones any more. Find what works to help your journey.

For women entering peri-menopause and those already in its throes the best management is understanding the physical, emotional and social changes – which is why I wrote this book. Information changes attitudes and increases acceptance. A UK intervention study found that women who completed an education program about menopause and learned what to expect reported fewer symptoms compared to women who did not receive the education. This is significant and reinforces the need to break the silence around menopause and increase the availability of information to enhance women's ability to cope.

Psychologists working with women during the menopausal transition report that many women identify a new sense of confidence. Menopause can bring the dawning of self-acceptance, an increased sense of self-worth and, importantly, less concern for how others may judge them. Psychologists also identify several issues that need to be addressed for women who may be struggling with menopause and age transition. Self-acceptance is crucial to aging well and this means understanding your strengths and weaknesses, but primarily focusing on using and building your strengths, and forgiving yourself your human failings. Better to know your genuine self and enjoy your real life than try and be something unsustainable like a superwoman – it is too exhausting, and that type of fatigue shortens your lifespan.

Another goal is to learn to treasure your physical body – after all, it has been your home and carried you around the earth. However, for some women body dissatisfaction is a real problem. It can be liberating not worrying about being perceived as sexually attractive to others or not, but rather focusing on satisfying one's own sense of attractiveness and becoming at home within one's skin. It may also save time and money!

The other body issue is where women are divorced from their physical selves and have limited knowledge about symptoms and body changes, as they have higher anxiety and often experience more symptoms. Again, being informed and developing body awareness and respect is very important. Treasure and care for your body home as you would your house.

Women's attitudes to other women matter and they change across the age span from puberty through fertile years and menopause. The most negative comments by women about women are given to women in menopause. Young women are the harshest critics, which would make mother–daughter relationships difficult for those in menopause who have teen or young adult daughters living at home. It would also be particularly difficult for young women experiencing early and premature menopause. For all our sakes, women must be kind to other women, and start telling a new, accepting and positive story about being female generally (being fertile is not a curse), and about menopause specifically as a time of transformation.

Developing self-confidence and a stronger identity is empowering and energising. Check your attitudes and channel your energies positively so you can grow.

Self-care: Develop a positive attitude

- **Embrace menopause.** Celebrate no more periods and that menopause means you have had reproductive health. Remember having to plan and prepare for periods, the cost of all those female hygiene products, ugly period underpants, changing your outfit, worrying about accidents and possibly cramping. It's all over, gone, finished. Say goodbye to pregnancy worry if you are heterosexual (and no longer needing contraception). Enjoy sex for sexual pleasure with no distraction of pregnancy risk.
- **Focus on your health.** Menopause is the perfect time and reason to prioritise your own health. Invest in your mental, physical, spiritual and emotional wellbeing and make changes to your lifestyle so you can age positively now and for the next thirty years.
- **Settle into your own skin.** Celebrate your wonderful lived-in body as it has got you this far. Understand and appreciate what your body can do for you – take on some new physical activities and enjoy developing new strength, fitness, coordination. Celebrate your own individuality and looks. Dress for yourself and not others and develop your own style. Happier, healthier and more confident is sexier, and let your uniqueness be your signature strength.
- **Find your voice.** Recognise your individuality and need for autonomy. Become assertive and defend your rights

while respecting other people's, and balance your needs with those of your family or significant others. Develop financial literacy so that you feel confident across all areas of your life, and do not be worn down or dissuaded from pursuing your goals.

- **Let your strengths shine.** Recognise your capabilities and strengths and stop hiding them or being self-deprecating. We need to know our strengths as we rely upon them to grow and solve problems. Be confident with what you think, know and can do and use your strengths as a basis for your goals.

- **Cultivate gratitude.** Consider all that you are grateful for – taking a moment each day to practise gratitude has major benefits. It may be tangible things, but there are greater mental and physical benefits to being grateful for people, places, experiences and health – anything that enriches us emotionally and spiritually.

- **Accept vulnerability.** If at all possible, stop caring for others at the expense of yourself. Perhaps learn to be vulnerable, ask for help and accept care too.

- **Follow your dreams.** You have several decades ahead of you and the wisdom and experience from the first half of your life to help you. Increase your sense of identity by doing more things for yourself and set about reaching those dreams that may have been put on hold. Stop wasting time. Find your passions and goals and set about making them happen.

- **Recruit support.** Share your female experience – talk to your women friends, share stories and build a closer supportive network. Seek professional help and appropriate treatment if you are struggling with mental health issues.

Summary: Caring for brain and mind

Women's sexual reproductive hormones are involved in brain health, brain function and emotion. Oestrogen is involved in cognitive functions such as memory and learning, as well as mood and mental health.

- **Boost brain health.** Your brain is your greatest asset so care for it by reducing brain burdens like stress, substance misuse and sleep disturbance. Build your brain's resilience by eating a nutritious diet, getting regular physical exercise and engaging in new and mentally stimulating activities.
- **Increase your experiences.** It is true that using your brain increases your cognitive capacity, so don't think about resigning or settling just yet. Expand your experiences and look outwards to new adventures and activities and find the joy in them. Remember what makes you feel good and repeat them to continually boost positive emotional experience. Perhaps pursue interests that you may previously not have had time for; take up a new hobby, join a club, find new friends. Get out into life.
- **Maintain mental wellbeing.** Check in regularly with yourself and manage stress as soon as it arises. You know your triggers and what your needs are so live according to your priorities and reduce your exposure to stress and undermining experiences. Liberate yourself from other people's expectations and follow your own dreams.
- **Cultivate a positive attitude.** Nurturing our wellbeing and revealing our best true selves are linked to improved health, longevity, lower risk of disability and considerably boosting quality of life. A positive attitude is also linked to increased self-awareness and stronger personal identity. A wonderful period for growth and contribution, this can be energising, liberating and positive when considered in the right light.

PART 5

SEX, RELATIONSHIPS AND ROLES

Humans are social and interdependent beings and are hardwired to have relationships for survival. The necessary neural pathways are laid down during our foetal development, augmented by hormones, and shaped by our early childhood experiences. Our intimate, family and social relationships, and our psychological needs from them, adapt and change across our lifespan. There are many internal and external factors that impact upon our relationships and roles.

Our reproductive hormones affect our motivation and behaviour and our roles shift in concert with those hormonal changes. Women have different roles across their lifespan related to their reproductive stage, such as the transition from being a pre-pubescent interested in friendships to a sexually fertile woman interested in sex and partnering. For those who have been pregnant you may recall the nesting drive prior to the birth of your child, which drove all sorts of behaviour such as spring cleaning, preparing the nursery and being acutely focused on your unborn child and much less on other people. These times of heightened interest and drive are due to the increase in the female sexual reproductive hormones.

The hormonal changes of menopause also significantly influence motivation and behaviour, including sex drive, feelings of nurturing, connection and intimacy. The last time during a woman's life cycle that her reproductive hormones were so profoundly changing her relationship behaviour was during puberty. Then, background life to that hormone chaos was relatively simple: school, home and socialising. In contrast the menopause transition occurs when women's lives are extremely complex as they have multiple relationships, roles and responsibilities. I call the complexity the menopause-midlife trifecta as women experience three simultaneous forces: changing hormones, increasing age and midlife-family stage.

For example, a woman in midlife entering the menopause transition is likely to be in a long-term relationship (or possibly recently separated, divorced or discovering a new partnership), have teenage or younger children living at home, be caring for older parents, be in employment, studying and/or volunteering, and have domestic, financial, family and social responsibilities. This may make navigating the menopausal transition difficult and any hormonal changes to motivation, behaviour and social-emotional connection can compound issues and have a significant impact on quality of life.

With so much going on, it can be difficult to distinguish the causes from the consequences. It may be easy to attribute alterations in sex and relationship dynamics to menopause, but it might not be the cause, as multiple other factors also play a role. Big-picture considerations are increasing age, general health, family stage, relationship quality and socio-environmental aspects. All relationship and role changes influence each other, and affect our sexual and emotional intimacy, feelings of connection and belonging, roles, priorities and meaning in life.

Sex and menopause

The menopause transition impacts upon sex drive, desire, function and satisfaction. Age also plays a role but the biological and psychological changes that occur in menopause are independently important, meaning that some changes are solely due to menopause and are unrelated to increasing age. Other influences on sex drive and desire include physical and/or mental illness, medication, relationship quality, psycho-social stressors, and situation or environment.

Sex drive is an evolutionary imperative but varies considerably between people. Sexual desire and drive is a highly complex area in women's health and are far more complicated than for males. Research indicates that sex drive and desire in biological males is relatively straightforward and that sexual issues are largely mechanical and not psychological. In contrast, sexual drive and desire in females involves biological, physiological and psychological factors. It is believed that this is due to the different outcomes of sexual reproduction for men and women. In heterosexual women sex, if successful in sexual reproductive terms, results in a nine-month pregnancy and years of parenthood. Therefore, to meet evolutionary requirements to have a successful pregnancy and to increase offspring survival, the female sex drive and desire has a lot of safety checks involved, including psychological factors such as a need for emotional connection and security, and these are largely driven by hormones.

Sex in humans, however, is not just for the evolutionary purpose of procreation. Sex and sexuality also provide a sense of pleasure, connection, increased emotional intimacy, and may enhance self-esteem and boost health. This means that after the sexual reproductive stage of a woman's life, sex and sexual intimacy may remain important.

Case study: Lost libido

I have found menopause a bit of a struggle emotionally. I turn sixty this year. The biggest impact upon me, as we can all deal with hot flushes, is the personal way I feel. My intimacy tap turned off completely and it's never been turned back on, which has been difficult. I love people but that intimacy with my husband is just gone. I was never that person.

It happened in the last five years. It is something to work really hard at and try overcoming but it's my biggest issue. No one talks about this. My husband noticed it, as it was such a big change, and he thought I didn't love him any more. I told him I didn't know what was happening, but I just couldn't go there any more. I would close my eyes and grit my teeth and that's not the point. I feel we have a great relationship, but the thought of sex makes my skin crawl. I can't understand how I've gone from loving sex and now, I can't stand the thought of it.

My husband is great, and he read everything he could. He is fantastic, quiet, patient and understanding. Our partners are such big players in taking away the guilt. I am lucky to have an amazing husband. We have a really good relationship – we hold hands, we cuddle, we talk and share everything. I love him dearly.

But there's guilt all the time and I get quite down and feel blue at times. I know some women have treatment for this, but I have had breast cancer, so I'm not prepared to take anything. Women need to remove the guilt and expectation.

I feel I have a great relationship and we enjoy each other's company and just hang out. People make jokes about not having sex for months and I feel guilty thinking how long it has been for us.

I would like to overcome this guilt and just accept that is a physical thing, not a feeling that you have towards your partner or husband. We need to understand what is important in a relationship and not feel guilty and understand that this is part of our journey.

I think women should share this story a bit more, so we can have more understanding and support. Menopause is important for women, but it should be equally important for their men.

If you are going through menopause and are not sharing this with your partner, how can you expect any sympathy? Your interest in sex wanes in menopause and you need your husband to understand. You need to share.

Sexual drive and desire

Drive and desire are sensitive to any changes in our female reproductive hormones. Drive is the biological component of desire, which also includes the psychological and motivational elements. In the context of a woman's entire reproductive lifespan, sex drive and desire change in response to menstrual cycle, oral contraception, pregnancy, post-partum state, breastfeeding, oophorectomy, hysterectomy and the menopausal transition.

Sex drive naturally declines with increasing age in both men and women. Biological sex drive is after all about reproduction and is very sensitive to age. This decline makes evolutionary sense: as fertility goes down and the risks of birth defects and failed pregnancies increase, the desire to procreate needs to go down too. When young, fit and healthy our biological drive is to reproduce. As we age our biological material (genes) also age and our biological drive to procreate diminishes accordingly. The hormonal aspect of declining sex drive in women is predominantly due to the loss of androgens, including testosterone.

As mentioned earlier, humans have sex for many reasons other than procreation and some additional ones are fun, communication, tension release, affirmation, comfort, to induce sleep, as an expression of love, to please a partner, to validate or confirm the relationship, as connection after a rupture in the relationship, and to relieve pain. This is where a hormonal change in drive and desire can become problematic. However, there are multiple additional physical, physiological, psychological and emotional factors that may increase or inhibit our desire for sex.

Science bite: Sex drive and desire

Drive and desire both impact the female body's physiological responsiveness to sexual activity, sexual function and satisfaction. Sex drive is a hormonally determined biological function of the brain and in women is associated primarily with oestrogen and androgens like testosterone. Drive is significantly influenced by desire. Desire encompasses biological sex drive as well as psychological, emotional relationships and individual aspects and relies more on oxytocin and dopamine. Sexual desire is a motivational state of interest in sexual activities and includes sex drive, feelings of trust and security, and pleasure.

Neuroscience research has revealed that we have three primary, discrete, interrelated emotion–motivation systems in the brain to support mating, reproduction and parenting: lust, attraction and male–female attachment. Each emotion–motivation system has evolved to fulfil specific roles to secure procreation, offspring and offspring survival. First is lust (sex drive) to initiate the search for a partner, followed by attraction so that we can make a selective choice and have sex with our preferred individual, and ending with attachment to enable prospective parents to work together and cooperate until parental duties have been completed.

Oestrogen impacts several organs and tissues that are involved in sexual arousal, physiological responsiveness and satisfaction including skin, breasts, muscles and urogenital organs. Loss of oestrogen therefore impacts sexual function and satisfaction as well as emotions associated with intimate connection such as trust and security as well as stress reactivity. Other physical menopausal symptoms such as weight gain, fatigue, hot flushes and night sweats may also impact desire, along with change in self-identity, sense of sensuality and sexuality and other psychological components.

Studies consistently report that sexual concerns during menopause are linked to marital/relationship satisfaction (addressed in the next section) and sexual function difficulties such as vaginal dryness. In terms of the impact of changing desire, women experiencing early, premature or medical menopause report more sexual issues than women going through natural menopause. The inference is that they experience more issues due to the abrupt cessation of hormones and lack of time for the body to physiologically adapt. However, those women also report lower relationship quality as well. Perhaps the difference between natural and medical menopause in terms of relationships and sexual issues is also due to the lack of time for psychological and emotional adjustment for women and possibly their partners too.

Changes in sexual desire and function are compounded by unhelpful messages about sex and sexuality. We live in an increasingly sexualised society and as a result the perception of what is normal is being skewed and there is increasing insecurity about sex drive and desire. More adults today think they may have a problematic loss of sexual drive and desire and/or are not having sexual intimacy at 'normal' levels. There is no normal level!

I reiterate: there is no standard or normal level of sex drive or desire. We all fall on a continuum from no drive to high drive and we each move along the range, or not, depending upon the multiple factors mentioned above (hormones, age, life stage, individual, psychological, relationship, situation or environment). If there is no normal, what makes a problem? Dissatisfaction – which is entirely subjective. Unless a person is dissatisfied with their sex life there is no problem, and a sexual dysfunction only exists if it causes *significant distress*. Not having sexual drive or sexual desire is not a problem unless you want to have sex drive and your lack of it causes you distress.

Previously, diagnoses of sexual dysfunctions were complicated and there were different types of disorders, but these have now been merged into a single condition called sexual interest/arousal disorder. The thought that sex might be nice, sometimes, but you can't be bothered, and not having sex is not a big deal, is not a sexual dysfunction. In fact, it is pretty common. A national investigation of Australian women in mid age found that 'low' desire was very prevalent – experienced by over sixty per cent of women. However, only thirty per cent reported significant distress because of their low desire and only they can be diagnosed with sexual interest/arousal disorder.

As a universal rule, if a person's level of desire and fulfilment is satisfactory and not causing distress for them and/or their partner, it is not a disorder. There are no models of female sexual desire; rather, it is complex and individual, and a bio-psycho-social, multidimensional and integrative perspective must be adopted in trying to understand it. Another important consideration is that sexual desire naturally changes, and not just with chronological age but relationship age and life stage too.

Sexual function

Aside from sex drive and desire, menopause also impacts on sexual function. Oestrogen during puberty increases vaginal lubrication and the 'plumpness' of the vaginal walls. During peri-menopause and menopause the lowering of oestrogen immediately impacts not only the vagina but the whole urogenital environment. The most commonly reported symptoms of urogenital deterioration are vaginal dryness, irritation and itching; they start with the onset of the menopause transition and are usually progressive in nature.

Often these symptoms get bundled together within the term genitourinary syndrome of menopause and includes the vulva, vagina and lower urinary tract. The vaginal walls become drier, thinner and less elastic. They also have a lower blood supply. The medical term is vaginal atrophy. Atrophic changes of the vulva, vagina and lower urinary tract can have a large impact on the lives of menopausal women. Along with vaginal dryness the vulva can also become dry and painful. The changes to the vaginal protective mucosa and loss of lubrication can lead to other symptoms of dryness and itching or burning, and painful intercourse. Other urogenital complaints include increased urinary frequency, stress-urinary incontinence and urinary tract infections.

These issues also make sex painful and functionally difficult. Sex that hurts in an unwanted way is not conducive to desire and a national study found that vaginal dryness and pain during or after sexual intercourse were significant factors contributing to low desire and sexual interest/arousal disorder. Painful intercourse can also make a woman fearful of pain and increase anxiety, which can burden mental health, and further reduce desire. Any increasing stress worsens many other symptoms of menopause and steals libido. Avoidance of all things sexual and sensual can result in a total loss of physical connection, and lead to distress, sometimes leading to a negative cycle, as these issues all worsen the likelihood of discomfort and reduce quality of life.

Although approximately fifty per cent of women experience these types of changes in their sexual lives only twenty-five per cent will seek medical or health advice. Ideally more women will begin to discuss sexual issues as there are plenty of hormonal and non-hormonal treatment options for urogenital discomfort and conditions. For example, vaginal dryness treatment options range from vaginal moisturisers, vaginal oestrogen applications, lubricants and oils, to consuming flaxseed in your diet and increased hydration, to stimulating regenerative treatments and hormone therapy. Find a sensitive and approachable doctor to discuss your sexual desire and function with as these issues can be treated. If not, they may negatively impact wellbeing, put stress on intimate relationships, and may reduce life satisfaction.

Science bite: Oestrogen, collagen, elastin and vaginal dryness

The reduction of oestrogen reduces elasticity and collagen throughout the entire body. For many women this significantly contributes to their aging process. The skin becomes less elastic and dry and loses its shape due to volume loss. The adverse effect on collagen synthesis also directly impacts vulvovaginal tissue and the growth of the vaginal epithelial lining. Multiple types of cells are affected which leads to vaginal atrophy. What you may notice is vaginal thinning, along with loss of vaginal lubrication – dry and pale mucus, itchiness, irritation and post-coital bleeding. These changes can be measured with the vaginal maturation value (VMV), which measures the amount of certain types of cells. Some women may also experience urinary tract issues such as urgency, frequency and recurrent urinary tract infections. Complete your pelvic floor exercises, keep hydrated, maintain cleanliness and pass urine after sexual activity. Seek professional help if required.

Case study: UK sojourn

I went through menopause between fifty and fifty-five, I think. I barely noticed it and the only symptom I had was noticing my libido was lower.

I took myself to the doctors, who prescribed testosterone and Vagifem. I did not use either as my husband thought it would pass and for him it was not an issue – he believed we still had a warm and emotionally intimate relationship and was not happy for me to take anything.

He believed the loss of libido was all to do with being in his mother's house while we were away, and he booked many weekends away to remedy the situation!

*I had no hot flushes, and no mood swings. Periods
became intermittent and then non-existent over a few
years – and when I had my yearly blood tests at I think age
fifty-five they confirmed I was post-menopausal.*

*I am happy to say, I barely noticed the change. I think
living in London and being very happy and busy, and
having a loving husband had a lot to do with it!*

Sexual satisfaction

Like sexual desire and function, sexual satisfaction also changes
with menopause and age, and also involves both physiological and
emotional response. During the menopause transition, hormone
changes decrease intensity of sexual orgasm and, in that sense,
may reduce physiological satisfaction, but emotional intimacy
needs may still be met.

Our bonding and social behaviour are influenced by oxytocin,
also known as the 'love hormone'. Oxytocin is both a hormone
and a neurotransmitter, which means it works within the brain
as well as influencing the body. Oxytocin is usually thought of as
a female hormone for lactation and levels do rise when women
give birth. However, oxytocin also impacts multiple areas of the
reproductive system and behaviour such as bonding, sex drive
and orgasm. During the menopausal transition, and afterwards,
the lowered levels of oestrogen reduce oxytocin production in the
brain and this can lower sexual satisfaction and/or relationship
satisfaction including feelings of security.

Orgasm stimulates oxytocin and has health benefits, not just
sexual and emotional ones. Orgasm is important to stimulate
blood flow, which helps protect the vaginal environment. There
are of course many ways to orgasm, but sexual intercourse or
sex is a matter for both or all people concerned, and changes in
desire, drive and satisfaction may need to be discussed within the

relationship. If penetrative sex becomes painful and/or stops being satisfying, consider *how* you have sex – it may be necessary to change or expand your repertoire. In youth one tends to have a diverse range of sexual practices and postures which decline with the duration of the relationship and increasing age. However, with menopause, injury, health conditions and age, new considerations for sexual pleasure may be necessary. Rather than intercourse with vaginal penetration, consider clitoral stimulation or oral sex. It may also be interesting to see if sex aids are helpful to increase pleasure and satisfaction. If there are differences in libido, masturbation may be a great way to maintain satisfaction without over-burdening the relationship.

It may be that you prioritise the snuggle-and-cuddle connection to express your emotional attachment, or to be very emotionally intimate. With any physical contact you will still get a burst of the 'cuddle' hormone oxytocin, just at a lower level than the burst at orgasm. Either way, we all significantly benefit from physical closeness, and the immediate physiological rewards of oxytocin include increased immunity and lower stress. The emotional benefits are limitless.

Conversations about sex and sexual satisfaction require a healthy positive relationship to support honest respectful communication, and such conversations will further build the depth and intimacy of the relationship. Changes in sex and intimacy can be very challenging and confronting for some couples as they may discover there is not enough emotional glue of kindness, respect, support and healthy communication between them, so seek professional relationship support and or sexual counselling if necessary

---

Science bite: Pelvic floor

The pelvic floor includes muscles, ligaments and connective tissues that support the pelvic organs – bladder, uterus, vagina and rectum – and acts like a sling or hammock supporting them in our body as well as helping them to function. When our pelvic floor muscles are contracted we lift those organs and the vagina, anus and urethra sphincters are tightened, which closes off their opening and stops urine or wind escaping.

Pelvic floor health is crucial for continence as well as sexual function. Pregnancies and childbirth, and surgeries such as fibroidectomies and hysterectomies, all stretch and/or weaken the pelvic floor. Menopausal changes to smooth muscles also affect it, along with activities that press downwards such as coughing, lifting heavy objects and straining to toilet. Pelvic floor exercises strengthen the pelvic floor. A weak pelvic floor results in incontinence, which is a serious issue for both men and women as they age. The more serious health condition is when a pelvic organ falls from its usual place and sags or bulges into the vagina. This is termed pelvic organ prolapse (POP), and surgery is usually necessary to repair it. Look online for pelvic floor exercises and discuss with your health practitioner.

Sexual inhibitors

Sexual inhibitors are those factors that reduce drive and desire and can be classified as physical, situational or environmental, psychological and relationship. Physical factors include general health, physical discomfort, pain, illness, disability, disease, medications and excess alcohol or recreational drug use, and the issues with female sexual function described above. Fatigue also reduces drive and desire. Often fatigue levels are related to family life stage. Peri-menopause usually starts when women are aged in their mid-forties, which often coincides with the busiest time of life and juggling multiple roles. Fatigue is a significant issue, not only because women are left exhausted but also because it increases cortisol and reduces androgens that are necessary for sex drive.

Physical factors also include the sexual function and physical health of partners. Male partners also experience changes to their libido and sexual function with increasing age. Their testosterone levels decline, leading to lower sex drive, and they also experience changes to their sexual function as their sexual reproductive capacity declines and sperm quality deteriorates. Approximately forty per cent of men over age forty experience erectile dysfunction (previously known as impotence); this increases to seventy per cent by age seventy. Men may take hormones to address their libido and medication to correct functional issues.

Women may also think to boost their libido. After natural menopause women continue to make some testosterone in the ovaries for approximately twelve years and this may or may not be enough – it is subjective. Testosterone replacement is increasingly offered as a treatment option for women concerned with having a lower libido. However, as desire is complex and involves psychological and relationship factors as well as hormonal ones, it is important to consider all factors before adding any hormones to your body. Because stress reduces androgens necessary for sexual desire and drive, stress reduction ought to be considered as one strategy to increase sexual desire.

The presence of teenagers or parents in the family home is probably the most significant situational or environmental factor that inhibits sexual desire. Other external passion killers include lack of time, lack of privacy, poor atmosphere and distractions. Competing activities such as hobbies, interests, social media and screen time do take a toll on desire and may also erode intimacy because proximity – being in the same physical space as your partner – is important along with attention, time and opportunity.

Opportunity also includes freedom from responsibilities such as work, house work and parenting.

In women psychological factors significantly increase or decrease sexual drive and desire. They include mental wellbeing, feelings about oneself in terms of confidence and attractiveness, how close and trusting we feel with our partner or partners, and what is sometimes termed our erotic script. Our erotic script is made up of thoughts, beliefs, past experiences and feelings about sex, sexuality and what an individual finds sexy or a turn on.

A turn off, or psychological sexual inhibitor, is fear of pregnancy and in this regard, menopause can be a profoundly positive and liberating time for women with male partners. However, it is possible to get pregnant during peri-menopause and the transition, and the fluctuating hormones and menstrual changes can make it difficult to know you are even ovulating. Wait until post-menopause before ceasing contraception.

Science bite: Fertility

Fertility is declining as we age, but it only takes one viable egg and one strong sperm. An irregular cycle can mean you are ovulating more than once per cycle. While the statistics indicate a very low two per cent chance of pregnancy for women aged between forty-five and forty-nine, that still means two women per hundred can become pregnant. After age fifty the chance is less than one woman per hundred. If you are in peri-menopause you still need to consider contraception, and the current recommendation is to continue to take contraception for two years after your last period. It is also crucial to discuss contraception as part of your menopause health management as there are different types of contraception available and they have different risks and implications for your menopause transition and longer-term health. Alternatively, use condoms or get your male partner/s to have a vasectomy.

Case study: Contraceptive pill

I went off the pill, after having been on it for many years, aged about forty-six when I (finally) was able to offload contraception responsibility – with the help of my husband having a vasectomy!

Pretty soon I started the throwing off and pulling on bed covers routine, but because I was 'young' I didn't click about pre-menopause. Periods were still happening but lighter and fewer ... all over the shop, which I put down to my body settling into its post-pill state.

It wasn't until I started having day-time 'flushes' that I even thought about menopause. I do clearly remember one day sitting in the car at traffic lights that had gone green and being tooted from behind because I SIMPLY HAD to instantly get off a jacket. I think for me, the term that seems to be used in American literature of 'hot FLASHES', as opposed to 'hot flushes', more accurately described that sudden un-ignorable temperature surge.

Nights were getting much worse – frequent dripping, wet nighties were the clincher – and I spoke with my doctor. We discussed various management options and I chose to go back onto a very low dose contraceptive pill. This absolutely did the trick – I had my bone density monitored, started on Caltrate and increased weight bearing and resistance exercise.

I continued on the pill for a few years until, in consultation with my doctor, I decided to go 'cold turkey' and see what happened. I had some easily ignorable minor overheating issues, which gradually receded. By the time I was forty-nine to fifty years old it was all over and I was 'through' menopause.

However, fear of pregnancy is a relatively minor consideration. The key psychological factors that impact drive and desire are levels of intimacy and relationship satisfaction. Intimacy is more complicated than sexual and physical connection with your partner, as it also comprises how you relate to yourself. The facets of intimacy include sexual, physical, emotional, spiritual and mental connection. As the expression states, 'You can't love another until you love yourself.' Intimacy is also associated with hormonally driven emotion–motivation factors such as security and trust, as well as feelings of love and attachment, and these are related to our relationships. Psychological factors are intertwined with relationship ones and research indicates that the most significant inhibitor of female sexual desire is the quality of their intimate relationships. The most effective way for women to improve their sexual desire is to improve the quality of their intimate relationships.

Self-care: Sex and sexuality

Caring for sexuality, in the same way we care for our physical health, is necessary for psychological wellbeing and quality of life. The important factor is to identify your individual needs and honour them.

- **Develop self-knowledge.** Identify what your sex drive and desires are – they are yours alone – and accept them. There is no problem unless there is concern. Consider your level of intimacy with your inner self – consider your physical, emotional, spiritual, mental and sexual connections. Then develop a plan to meet all those aspects.
- **Explore.** Try out new sexual behaviours. Rather than intercourse try outer-course or use sex aids. Cuddles, massage and other forms of physical contact may be pleasurable and intimate. Consider expanding your

195

repertoire to have new languages of love – sharing interests, spending time together, building dreams, starting new projects and activities, and doing things for each other.

- **Investigate**. There are lots of different treatment options for sexual function difficulties – local ones such as lubricants that act specifically on the area, or systemic ones that impact the whole body – so enquire and conduct your own research until you find what suits your and your partner's needs.
- **Communicate**. Talk honestly with your partner/s about how you are feeling – emotionally, physically, psychologically – and discuss your drive and desire. Listen to their experiences too. Talk through desire discrepancy and perhaps separate sex from love. Find a mutually satisfactory solution and keep communicating, as needs change with time and age.
- **Consult a professional**. There are many health professionals you can discuss these issues with, from your GP to a psychologist, sexual counsellor, marriage counsellor or medical specialist such as a gynaecologist.

Intimate relationships

Our needs from our intimate relationships change over our reproductive life and lifespan. Qualitative studies of women in the menopause transition indicate that multiple psycho-social variables combine to help shape their relationship experience. The studies indicate that while menopause is an important milestone in women's development it may have less impact on women's health and happiness than their intimate relationships. Multiple fields of medicine and psychology confirm that good-quality relationships are crucial to women's health and wellbeing, and for many their intimate relationship/s is/are what they value most in life.

Relationship quality can either contribute to or diminish a woman's capacity to cope with all aspects of life, including significant health challenges and menopause. For example, research indicates that a supportive relationship buffers, or reduces, the negative impact of breast cancer, and increases adjustment and coping.

Relationship quality includes level of attraction to a partner and level of intimacy (physical, emotional, spiritual, mental and sexual), and trust, security, communication, respect, unresolved conflict, sexual expression and age of relationship. These factors have more impact on desire than menopause, but menopause is often blamed for its diminishment.

The difference between the women who are, and are not, concerned about the change in their sex lives is largely due to their relationship status, quality and stage, and their different attitudes towards sex and relationships. This is distinct from menopausal stage as sexual satisfaction has been found to be directly related to relationship satisfaction and not menopause status. It is important to note that in these studies sexual satisfaction was not defined as sexual intercourse but as satisfaction with how sexuality was expressed within the relationship. For most women changes in their sex life are not a significant issue at all. A change in libido due to menopause causes only a minority of women significant concern. Those women who do report increased relationship stress due to their sexual changes also report general relationship problems, as the two are linked. They also report greater sleep difficulties and increased stress related to marital problems, as low relationship quality has been found to increase menopause symptoms and general stress-related health issues.

Level of support impacts relationship quality, and feeling unsupported is a factor that significantly inhibits desire. Research suggests that an increase in the quality of emotional intimacy within the relationship and increased domestic support from one's partner/s increases desire. When you consider how fatigue impacts the hormones of sex drive, it is obvious how domestic support can be helpful in multiple ways.

Relationship stage or longevity also impacts desire but not necessarily quality. Studies suggest that over the course of a long-term partnership sexual intimacy between partners changes as does its meaning and importance in the relationship. Being with the same partner for a long time can diminish sexual intimacy, because familiarity can divest relationships of sexual energy. But plenty of long-term couples who have significantly decreased sexual intimacy report high relationship satisfaction, because they are high on other forms of intimacy. This is where it is important to ignore external societal messages about sex and instead focus in on all areas of intimacy and the nature and quality of your relationship.

Menopause puts a spotlight on intimate relationships and may be a profound trigger for change. The menopause transition does not necessarily *cause* these changes, but the biological drive to partner for sex or procreation diminishes and some relationships can become unstuck if there are insufficient or inadequate alternative ties. After the sex-reproductive phase of their lives women increasingly focus on other forms of intimacy, and if these are lacking the relationship becomes unsatisfactory. Interestingly, within Chinese medicine, menopause is perceived as a shift of energy from the womb to the heart centre, complementing the shift from sexual intimacy to other forms of connection, energy and love.

In one study, over two hundred women were questioned regarding their marriage, stress and menopause and their responses indicated an unsatisfying marriage left women more vulnerable to stress and they had more menopause symptoms than those in satisfying relationships. Symptoms such as sleep disturbance and hot flushes were also found to be worse in the context of a dissatisfactory relationship. An unsatisfying marriage was characterised by less domestic and childcare support, less emotional intimacy and higher conflict.

The hormone rewiring of menopause that affects the biological drive and motivation towards sex and bonding behaviour supports a relationship review. Without biological drives influencing behaviour, women are free to evaluate their intimate relationships in terms of other factors such as level of emotional intimacy, support, shared interests and trust. Relationships at the early stage are often characterised by joint projects such as building a home, raising children, supporting careers and establishing financial security. These types of relationships are called transactional, as partners are involved in transacting goods/services and have reciprocal expectations. For both men and women, bonding for procreation and to raise children is a transactional exchange.

With increasing age, and menopause, the relationship focus shifts to more related connection and transformational enrichment. Studies suggest that this increases desire for companionship and intimacy, and requires reconsiderations for support, companionship, equality, shared interests, co-partnership, complementary or support for future dreams as well as self-development. Finding your own voice and becoming confident in your own skin (self-intimacy), as distinct from your partner/s, is an important psychological developmental task of adulthood and a supportive high-quality relationship will help you to get there.

The pressures upon intimate relationships that coincide with the menopause transition may in fact be due to midlife and/or family-life stage. The influences include stagnation, changes in priority and purpose in life, inequity and lack of support, fatigue, and longer-term relationships that may have become tired, stale or past their use-by date. Importantly the influence of external factors on psychological resilience changes depending upon stage of menopause. For example, financial stress impacts sexual desire in women during the menopause transition but not for women pre- or post-menopause. This suggests that during the transition, women, especially those in low-quality relationships, are more susceptible to the negative impact of external stressors.

Becoming and remaining well partnered takes time and effort but bestows multiple benefits. Unfortunately, the corollary is also true. People in unhealthy, unhappy or unsatisfying relationships have reduced health, lower quality of life and shorter lifespans. Being unhappy in a relationship is more detrimental than being single, divorced or widowed. It is important, then, that women look at their relationships and consider if they are enhancing or handicapping their wellbeing, and then sort out the best way to remedy the situation.

Case study: Secrets

I determined I would be more stoic than my mother when menopause came and was on full alert for the slightest change from my fiftieth birthday. I was peri-menopausal and having tidal wave periods until I was fifty-four. They were so heavy I was beginning to look forward to menopause. When my periods stopped for three months I couldn't have been happier.

At fifty-five I'm still getting period pains but no periods. I put on five kilos in no short order and found I became quite low. I felt like I was looking out through a haze of grey and nothing was right with the world. This lasted three months and simply stopped.

I braced myself for the battle my mother went through but so far it hasn't arrived. Even my doctor is a little amazed. I'm still waiting but at this point believe I may be one of the lucky ones who might ride through this more easily than most.

There was one startling self-realisation which I hadn't expected. I didn't tell my husband a thing about it. The idea

he might view me as old has kept me from doing this. Mad,
right? He can see more clearly than me my aging process.
I eventually put that right by talking with him, but I guess
no matter how far down life's road we go, a good dollop of
vanity and insecurity can hold us back from truly sharing
life with another.

The attitude of partners towards age and menopause is also very important and affects women's experience of the transition. Support and emotional empathy increase relationship satisfaction and positively impact the menopause experience. However, as indicated in the case study 'Secrets' above and the literature, most women do not in fact talk about their menopause experiences, either to their partners, friends or family. For example, despite how common hot flushes are and how debilitating they can be – especially those that last up to an hour – very few women will tell the people they are with that they are experiencing a flush.

This lack of disclosure increases any sense of isolation they feel within their relationship and may threaten relationship satisfaction. Additionally, for some women, and especially if their partner celebrates youthfulness over uniqueness, menopause can increase a sense of vulnerability and insecurity within the relationship. Fear or insecurity within a relationship has profound impacts on a woman's confidence, desire, wellbeing and relationship satisfaction. The fear of being replaced by a younger version is not irrational. I know a woman who is older than her husband and is terrified about what her menopause may mean for her relationship. She has lost her sex drive and desire, put on some extra weight, and lost confidence in her sexual attractiveness – she is terrified her husband will be unfaithful and start a relationship with a younger woman. The statistics confirm that midlife relationship breakdown is very common, and reasonable numbers of midlife men do commence new relationships with younger women.

We need to have open conversations about the menopause experience with our partners to garner their support. Remember your partner may know you well but he is not a mind-reader and can't see inside your body to know what is happening. Break the silence and share with your partner what you are experiencing, your concerns, expectations, and how you want to be best supported by him. The transition lasts a long time and is a significant time in your life. If your partner is not interested in your wellbeing and in being supportive, then a relationship review is clearly necessary.

Case study: Murderous menopause

My period stopped for about six months, then came back for a couple of months. My final period ended just like my first period. Extremely heavy with large clotting – I sat around the bathroom for two days. It finished, and I never had another. I must say I have never missed them.

I felt my mood change before my periods stopped; I went to my GP as I felt I was going 'crazy' so he did some blood tests, but they came back normal. However, he did say women feel menopause before the tests come back with evidence.

My life and marriage were good enough. But I was getting angrier by the day; I felt I was losing my mind some days as I could not think straight. I remember one morning I got up out of bed and said to my husband and son, 'I'm feeling so angry today I feel I could kill.' They both looked at me and left, coming home that night.

Most mornings I would wake and be on my own as my husband worked away. I would be at home feeling like a crazy lady. Depression went with the anger. I wrote down my feelings when in a depressed state and this is what I wrote: Standing on the cliff edge, looking down, pondering the actual death of my soul, my being. But the threads are holding me back, the few threads of joy and love. The pain is so deep within my veins; my soul doesn't ever have peace. I get submerged in giving, pleasing and listening to my guilt-ridden conscience.

I recognised the lack of support and loneliness I felt in my marriage and got divorced.

Evidence supports addressing an unsatisfying relationship sooner rather than later. It is possible to be in a relationship and be lonely, and loneliness is a negative health burden linked to increased mental distress and mental illness as well as lowered immunity and increased morbidity and mortality. Do not delay a relationship rescue or considering your exit, for example, by waiting until the children leave home. Consider acting now while you have plenty of years and good health ahead with which to grow and reinvest. The risks of not improving intimate relationships jeopardises women's health. The stress associated with remaining in unsatisfying relationships directly impacts the menopause transition and the three post-menopause diseases, cardiovascular disease, breast cancer and depression, and shortens women's lifespans. Now is the time for women to be the people they want to be, rather than being who they think their partners want, and to live and love accordingly.

Self-care: Invest in relationships

A review of relationship status during the transition can provide women with the opportunity to rediscover themselves as individuals and as a part of a couple. Consider your (shared) history but focus on your needs for intimacy and what type of relationship you want in your future.

- **Getting connected.** For singles who want to be connected, how you think about menopause may either energise you or de-energise you. Start with your mindstyle. Becoming attached is going to be tough as the numbers are stacked against you – there are more women than men. Celebrate your uniqueness and life experience. You do not need a makeover or plastic surgery to look younger; instead, honour yourself and build confidence, which is attractive and sexy, and do not let a man's lack of interest and appreciation become your concern – it reflects them not you. As stated by a Boomer male, there is nothing sadder than an older guy with the emotional depth of a teenager trying to date a younger woman. Live your life for you.

- **Reconnect (or disconnect).** Confirm the good qualities in your relationship and those of your partner. It is easy to see fault and take the good for granted, especially if the relationship is long term and feeling stale. Reflect on the qualities that made you fall in love – are they still there? Find your own identity and voice and see if the relationship can adjust and grow with the new empowered you. If not, fly solo to bloom, and give yourself the opportunity, if you want to re-partner. Part company respectfully in recognition that the relationship is no longer satisfying and health enhancing but perhaps once was.

- **Build companionship.** From midlife we move into a more companionship-oriented stage in our relationships from a transactional one. Have a second honeymoon, arrange date nights, revisit favourite haunts, go on adventures and discover new things together. Singles, get busy creating an active life without a partner and enjoy lifelong sustaining friendships. Appreciate the difference between being alone and being lonely in a relationship.

- **Communicate.** Keep the communication open and respectful. Stop thinking you are a mind-reader, or assuming you know, and ask your partner/s and friends for their thoughts, feelings and expectations instead. Developing healthy communication also allows you to manage threats to relationships such as accumulated daily stresses. Take responsibility for yourself only and reciprocate listening, truly hearing your partner without judgement.

- **Share dreams.** Keep developing shared goals and build plans together within intimate relationships, or with others of similar mind. Joint projects change over time so be sure you always have at least one shared interest or touch point at all times. Shared experiences and positive time together become the glue in relationships and strengthen resilience and team building for when times get tough. Having fun and sharing the joys of life boosts health and mental wellbeing.

- **Love is a verb.** To love means action. For those in a relationship consider how you demonstrate love, and how your partner displays love to you. There are different ways to communicate love to another person so ensure you are speaking the same language as your partner. (To learn more, read books by Dr Gary Chapman.) If you choose to be in a relationship appreciate your partner, keep seeing their positive qualities and attributes rather than focusing on the negative, and celebrate the good between you.

Maternal feelings

Maternal feelings are linked to caring and loving actions typically associated with caring and raising young. When women reach their sexual reproductive maturity their maternal drive has also developed so they have feelings and care behaviour necessary to look after any young that they may have. Maternal feelings are further increased during pregnancy and lactation. Maternal behaviour is therefore very sensitive to female hormones, with environment–context and experience also playing a role.

Animal studies confirm the complexity of maternal drive and behaviour and suggest that hormones and multiple structural areas of the brain are involved. The primary hormones that support maternal feelings of attachment, trust and motivation to care and bond are oestrogen, oxytocin and dopamine. Due to brain plasticity, involvement or engagement with babies and/or young children at a young age also positively influences the development of the maternal brain. Such exposure in women leads to their developing greater sensitivity to oxytocin, which translates to heightened maternal feelings and motivation. For example, I spent a great deal of my childhood babysitting younger cousins and the more I was engaged with their care the more I was motivated to have my own children and care for others.

Level of maternal drive varies between women. Approximately fifty per cent of women have children and they may or may not have strong maternal drive. For some women their maternal-care drive may have been directed towards pets, other people or other care projects, or into their careers or volunteering.

During the menopausal transition, maternal drive declines, as levels of oxytocin are related to levels of oestrogen. As a result, there is less hormonally driven behaviour towards caring and nurturing and this affects the carer–dependent relationships women may have. Additionally, the hormonal changes also influence feelings of affiliative need, which means getting on with others, and feelings of connection, which further impacts all relationships. It is not uncommon for many women to become selective about their friendships, focusing on quality over quantity.

The drop in the evolutionary drive to care and nurture may have a big impact, with some women feeling less inclined to cope with and tolerate the care demands of others. I know of a single woman whose two pet dogs were her much-loved child substitutes and clearly adored. When she entered the menopause transition her dogs were old and she decided they would not be replaced when they died so she could be 'free'. She planned a career sabbatical with a year of world travel. She did not want to be a pet carer any more but wanted to grow and expand her life experience.

This menopausal hormone-related change and the resulting feelings of diminished maternal caring are seldom discussed. This is in part due to the messaging around women as carers and the stigma of having low levels of maternal drive. As a result, the experience of lower levels of compulsive caring can leave some women feeling confused, guilty and ashamed. Some may no longer recognise themselves and wonder where their ambivalent feelings come from. However, it is important to appreciate that the reduction in maternal drive does not mean a diminishment of love; it simply means there is a reduction in the drive to care and provide for others and this is a natural shift.

To meet the changing demands of offspring, as well as threats to their survival, maternal behaviour has evolved to be very dynamic and flexible to change. All youth at some stage need to develop sufficient autonomy and capacity to self-care so that they can reproduce themselves. Human children are exceedingly dependent when born and remain dependent for a prolonged period compared to most large mammals. The level of nurturing they require needs to change to complement their developmental requirements. During menopause the reduction in mothering behaviour enables children the space and opportunity to grow into capable independent adults. Due to changes in the life cycle the timing of menopause and stage of child development has shifted. Previously menopause occurred when children were adults and had left the family home. Today adolescence has been extended into young adulthood, with young people being dependent and living at home for a much longer time than previous generations. This has a significant impact upon family structure and life-stage roles, and the menopause experience.

While maternal behaviour has evolved to be flexible and dynamic, if you have young people at home still relying upon you and the menopause transition starts to diminish the drive to care, flexibility may not be enough! Going through your own hormonal changes and simultaneously negotiating the hormonal and life-stage changes of teenagers and young adults can be very challenging. Add in menopausal symptoms of poor sleep, night flushes and/or increased stress and there may be significant risks to relationships and wellbeing. The combination of a change in women's biologically driven nurturing and teenagers' drive for independence can increase the risk of disharmony and disconnection between two opposing forces.

During a workshop on menopause it became clear that women with teenagers had significant difficulty managing the transition as they were simultaneously balancing the needs and demands of their child-adults. Internally they felt an increase in emotional reactivity and stress, which was usually manageable, but when the external forces of managing the social and emotional complexity of teenagers came along they were overwhelmed. A lack of support from partners exacerbates this situation, as highlighted in the previous section on the importance of healthy positive intimate relationships. The life-stage transition for parents and their children entering adulthood can be challenging for all family members and relationship dynamics, and sometimes things do not go to the original plan.

Case study: Detachment

I started having these episodes when I would become terribly down and feel incredibly isolated and dislocated from my family. I felt underappreciated, unloved, and that my husband and children did not know the real me and were not even interested. I felt lost in service to them and their needs, and resentful, as I didn't feel I wanted to be a mother/ housewife any more. Now that may sound familiar to lots of women with teenagers and a busy husband, especially one away a lot with work, but the difference was that after a few episodes I noticed a pattern!

I was in peri-menopause. It took me about four of these episodes to realise these unbearable feelings of disconnection and resentment were happening just before my periods. I felt so embarrassed, especially as I had never had PMS or mood swings before, and then, I felt ashamed. I adore my family.

Forever trying to be a good parent and wife, I thought I would be able to manage better the next time. That I would notice the feelings start and I would be able to stop myself criticising them for taking me for granted and not being helpful, or keep from succumbing to the sense of disconnection and guilt afterwards. It has taken me several years and I am not sure I have beaten it, but I reconfirm every day that I love them.

I know of several women who left their families during their menopausal transition as they could not sustain the care demands upon them. They were carers of their children and also their husbands and the lack of reciprocal care and emotional equity was draining them. They were giving out too much of their energy, time and care and it was not sustainable or reconcilable with their own needs. When I consider the type of relationships and family dynamics they left and the new relationships they have now forged, it is very clear that they needed to rebalance equity in care and support. They were able to reforge new adult relationships with their adult children and re-partner in more intimate and satisfying ways. Although these cases may appear extreme they are a good reminder of the importance of communication within relationships, as well as care, respect and positive patterns of relating. I know of other women who have felt energised to grow and redirect their energy, and who experienced a reduction of desire to care and be in service to their family members, but who have been able to navigate this change positively due to high-quality intimate relationships with their partners and good communication with their children.

Menopause may coincide with the time of 'empty nest', when children leave the family home to go on to tertiary study or their own adventures. The thought of having no dependents at home is exciting for some women – a time of growth, an opportunity to reconnect with partners, or take on new roles or embark on entirely new adventures. For other women it may be a time of grief and loss. There are several reasons why children leaving the family home can be a negative experience for some parents, in addition to the immediate absence of companionship and social interaction. Parents may be left feeling purposeless and redundant as the primary joint purpose of the union, to raise children, is over, or at least the requirements have profoundly changed. If you've built your identity on this role or project, who are you now? How do you fill your time? Marital conflicts may arise, and as there is less distraction from your intimate relationship and how you interrelate, any weaknesses will become increasingly obvious.

Moving forwards into the next stage of life means letting go of something so you can embark on something new. Letting go of compulsive care and the habit of self-sacrifice can also create loss, even if in the longer term it helps you to restore a new equitable balance and allows you more time to pursue your own goals. For those who have made maintenance of the family home their vocation, downsizing or change in this area can cause yet more grief. The heightened emotionality of menopause, changes in feelings of connection, and lower maternal drive may further contribute to feelings of loss. But we begin from endings, so it is important to understand loss as part of the natural process of change that allows growth.

As women fall along a continuum of maternal drive, each of us will experience the change in maternal feelings and empty nest differently. Some women will be acutely aware of the reduction in their feelings of caring while others may be unaware, and some but not all women will experience loss when children become adults and no longer need mothering.

The change from biological drive to care, however, provides a perfect opportunity for conscious choice to care and nurture those whom you choose to love, and/or rechannel that energy into yourself and new dreams. As maternal feelings diminish many women experience a surge of energy and a drive for self-fulfilment in new ways. Let go feelings of guilt or shame regarding changes in feelings of maternal care. Cultivate a kind loving inner voice, increase self-acceptance and refocus your energy in new ways. Refer to Part 4, Attitude, for more information.

Self-care: Redefine roles

- **Give love.** The best way to feel love is to love. Start with yourself. Learn to love yourself. Separate love from domestic responsibilities and the transactional elements of relationships from your love, so you can find the joy within each relationship rather than losing love in service functions.

- **Be vulnerable.** Allow others to care for you. Make caring and nurturing behaviour normal for all family members so everyone can give and receive. Develop equality and mutual responsibility and be mindful of your boundaries and honouring yourself as your own person with the same rights as others, and enable others to have the same rights.
- **Renegotiate roles.** Perhaps your children are old enough for more independence and to take on more responsibilities. Match your mothering care to their age and stage of maturity. It is important to support their domestic skill development and autonomy, so they can become independent adults. At age eighteen children are considered adults, so they need the life skills to support themselves, such as being able to cook, clean the entire house, manage their finances and pay at least part of their own way, wash and maintain their clothes and linen, and complete other domestic tasks. Consider graduated domestic and life-management tasks they can perform so you both can enjoy more positive time being together rather than doing things for them. Make plans to spend time together and develop shared interests.
- **Appreciate.** Focus on the good and reward positive behaviour rather than just picking up on the negative – yours and theirs. Give praise generously and make time to celebrate each member of the family. Treasure each other. Establish habits that involve quality time together such as a regular family meal, build shared interests, and take holidays or time out together.
- **Manage empty-nest sadness.** You know your children will leave eventually so start increasing non-parental interests and activities before it happens. Accept and celebrate their departure as it usually means you have done a great job – they are skilled and capable and feel independent

and autonomous, which is a huge achievement for them and you! Get involved in their successful transition by setting up regular contacts to stay in touch, such as weekly meals together. Extend your experiences by pursuing new interests and hobbies. Re-energise your intimate relationship – take a second honeymoon and rediscover yourselves as partners not parents.

- **Be flexible.** Ways of relating and communicating love may need to change and might take time for adjustment. It would be easier for all family members if it was understood that the menopause reduction in maternal behaviour does not mean a change in love, only in how love is demonstrated. Find a new balance between loving, caring and nurturing others and caring and nurturing yourself.
- **Redirect nurturing.** Women in midlife make up the majority of people advocating human rights and environmental protection measures to improve the planet and communities and to ensure a better life for the next generation. Redirect or rechannel your care and nurturing drive. Consider what causes are important to you and get involved. What is your legacy going to be?

Role transitions

There are generational differences in the life experiences of women and the roles they fulfil. The lifespan has extended significantly, and we have better health. Women today are out of the family home and in the public arena – through employment, social connection, care roles and other activities – more than previous generations. While this is obviously a positive sign of progress, it can make it harder to manage menopause symptoms and navigate the transition years.

Changes in our reproductive life cycle are now less likely to coincide with complementary lifespan changes. The complexity of our lives today has significant implications for how we experience and manage menopause, but also underscores the importance of resetting our health priorities.

Case study: Life stuff

I don't remember any 'psychological' issues for me during menopause. I certainly had no intention of having any more babies and I had always found periods to be a practical nuisance, so I was happy to be free from them. Being on the pill tended to mean it was difficult for me to lose weight, so once I stopped the pill and let menopause happen, I was able to more easily drop some of the extra weight I was carrying. If anything, I think I felt better about my physical self.

I find it difficult to say whether my general stress levels were affected by menopause. For me, and I suspect for many women, the timing of peri-menopause and actual menopause coincided with so much other 'stuff' going on in my life. Family things, and in particular some pretty significant issues with my son, and never-ending work issues related to the complexity of running a small business and employing staff, and the gradual morphing of friendships as time and circumstances change etc.

In my mind menopause wasn't really a 'big deal' in the scheme of things. I tend to be quite pragmatic about the normal processes and progressions of life. Maybe, for me, the significance of other 'life stuff' just overshadowed my menopause.

There are no neat bookend dates classifying each generation, but it is generally accepted that Boomers are those born between the end of WWII and the mid-sixties while those born after them up until the early eighties are called Generation X. Boomers are now aged from fifty-five to seventy-four and will either still be in the throes of menopause or long emerged out the other side. Generation X is the cohort now in or about to enter the menopausal transition.

The first wave of Boomer women turned eighteen in the mid-sixties and entered what has been called the sexual revolution, with the development of the contraceptive pill and hormone therapy. It was a time of significant economic growth and high employment, with individuals enjoying increased socioeconomic health and financial security. Many women in this group went to university or studied, for example, nursing or teaching, and entered the workforce but left to become mothers and the primary home manager and had their first child before age twenty-five. Divorce rates are very high for this cohort, and many women completed degrees in their midlife or late life, often post-divorce, and took on careers once their children left home. Unlike any generation before or after them, Boomer women have enjoyed unprecedented buying power and financial reserves, and their quality of life is rated as very high.

For Generation X there is a paradox. While on many measures life has improved for this group of women, with increased education, professional employment and some reduction of the gender wage gap, their overall wellbeing and life satisfaction has gone down. Their wellbeing has gone down relative to Generation X men's wellbeing, and it's gone down compared to Boomer women. There are many potential factors contributing to the lower level of life satisfaction of Generation X women, whose experiences are often characterised by a sense of exhaustion and stress. Not a good foundation before entering menopause.

Generation X women were told 'you can have it all' and 'you can do whatever you want', and as a result this generation thought the world had done a better job of catching up with the theory of equal rights than it actually has. The increase in their educational and occupational opportunities has not been matched with men's contributions at home. The lives of their male partners essentially remained the same as those led by the men of previous generations. There has not been help at a societal level either with wage equality, and added to this is a lack of adequate affordable childcare, and in some instances penalising tax measures. This has meant that Generation X women are often well educated, have careers and simultaneously continue to perform the lion's share of child-raising, domestic management and care roles.

The other difference for this generation is that while women today may earn more money than the previous generation of women, they have larger debts due to education fees, childcare costs and higher mortgages relative to income (if they can afford a home of their own at all), which for many women simply means they can't afford to stop work and have child-rearing as a primary focus if they want to, and are locked into simultaneous and often competing roles as workers and mothers. Generation X women won't retire when their parents did due to financial reasons, predominantly a lack of savings, and the age of retirement being extended. They are financially responsible for their children for much longer and this too depletes their financial security. The fact their children often remain at home longer may also deplete their emotional energy.

Another difference contributing to fatigue is that, unlike previous generations, Generation X, and late Boomers, are caught caring for their children and elderly parents at the same time. Previously there has been a two-step care process with a gap in between: raise children, (meno) pause, then care for parents; now it is part of the simultaneous juggle. Family care givers are predominantly female aged forty-nine, and for those who have children their eldest child on average is aged nineteen and most likely living at home. For this reason, Generation X is often termed the sandwich generation, as they are caught between two larger generation cohorts and being carers of both.

Generation X, and the last Boomers, may have had plenty of opportunities, but they also shoulder many simultaneous burdens that may contribute to a sense of exhaustion, compromise health and disempower them before the menopause transition even starts.

Navigating menopause at work

More women are now in employment and more are entering employment in their midlife to late life than ever before. This shift is due to economic and population changes, including a shrinking, aging workforce, as well as welcome societal progress. As a result, almost one quarter of the Australian workforce comprises women of menopausal age, which means they will be transitioning through menopause while in work. The silence around menopause in society is not helpful generally, but in the workplace it is a significant problem. We spend so much of our lives at work and need it to be a quality experience or risk our physical and mental health. Work affects our menopause experience, while menopause affects work productivity and has significant economic impact.

Economic and workplace productivity studies suggest that menopausal symptoms, vasomotor symptoms of hot flushes in particular, have a big impact on women at work. A large American study of a quarter of a million women with menopause symptoms found that unmanaged hot flushes in the workplace cost $370,000 over one year. Other work-impacting symptoms reported by women include headaches, sleep disturbance, weakness, fatigue and anxiety. Research also suggests that the workplace can make a profound difference to the menopause experience at work and reduce the potential cost burden. Yet international and local research indicates that most companies are not addressing this issue.

A UK investigation, for example, identified that only two per cent of employers had menopause as part of their occupational health and safety considerations and only twenty per cent of employers provided information about menopause to their employees.

Menopausal women in the workforce may worry about the intrusion of symptoms into their roles and work quality and feel stressed and anxious at work because of this, which has been found to lead to feelings of lower self-esteem and loss of confidence. Women report less job satisfaction, greater intention to leave, less engagement with work and less organisation commitment; however, less than one per cent reported having management training in awareness of menopause at work. Although the experience of women varies, a publication by the British Occupational Health Research Foundation entitled 'Women's Experience of Working through the Menopause' reported that nearly half of employed women found it somewhat or fairly difficult to cope with work during menopause. That is a lot of women.

The lack of employer support is a significant contributory factor. The secondary consequences of lack of support are a worsening of symptoms and further lowering of work productivity and confidence. There is also the effect of cognitive symptoms, such as loss of concentration and focus, and memory lapses that undermine confidence and impact performance. Some studies suggest that women in employment experience fewer physical symptoms than their non-employed counterparts. However, the same study indicates they experience more psychological issues, and that psycho-social workplace factors such as work stress and perceptions of control/autonomy and support influence the relationship between symptoms and work.

Various sources identify key areas where employers and organisations can improve the experience of women during the transition by addressing those features of the workplace that make symptoms worse, such as hot and poorly ventilated work environments, long formal meetings and high-visibility work – formal presentations where a woman experiencing a hot flush may be embarrassed and feel that her professional image may be compromised. Additional concerns were that women often worked extremely hard to overcome their perceived shortcomings and refrained from disclosing their concerns with managers even when taking time off work to manage their symptoms. One UK study reported that forty per cent of post-menopausal women felt their symptoms affected their work performance. The symptoms they believed to be compromising their work were trouble concentrating, tiredness, poor memory, depression, low confidence and sleep disturbance. This was a subjective report by women, so it would be interesting to know if there was any objective evidence of change in their work performance, as the data may reflect women being overly critical of themselves.

Case study: Executive plea

Working while going through menopause has to be addressed. Workplaces are shifting. We are helping workplaces change to support career optimisation rather than trying to change people, which is great for helping women. It is OK to talk about pregnancy or about age or about parent care, but we still can't talk about menopause.

We now have paternal leave, not just maternal leave. We also have carer's leave and assistance to help workers care for elderly parents. But what about menopause?

Pregnancy takes a huge toll on women's careers, but menopause takes even longer. Menopause affects women's performance. For example, I gave a presentation last week and would rate myself a 6.5 when I am usually a 9. My energy was so low because I had not slept since I have two to three night sweats every night and hot flushes during the day. My productivity is lower. I am so exhausted and struggling at work.

We have got to have this conversation about menopause in the workforce.

In 2018 menopause was described as the 'silent career killer'. Studies identified that menopause was linked to increased absenteeism, increased work dissatisfaction and increased doubt regarding one's job and employment. Given the statistics regarding the numbers of women of menopausal age in the workforce, their careers and the impact on the economy, support to improve women's work experience and occupational health during the transition must be developed. Work adjustments to manage workload, symptoms and productivity need to occur.

However, there remains a typically silent response in organisational contexts, which is related to the broader cultural suppression of women's health and reproductive journeys, as discussed in the introduction. There have been considerable improvements regarding maternal health and maternity leave, but menopause remains a taboo.

Some researchers suggest that the silence around menopause may also be a form of 'gendered ageism', an extension of older women being invisible in society generally and in workplaces specifically. As a result older women are often marginalised and overlooked in employment settings. The first bias is that women in their sexual reproductive years will leave to have babies, and after a certain age that they are too old. Women of menopausal age or post-menopause are less likely to have their employer support further job training or promotion due to concerns for their older age, imminent retirement and possible health issues.

Limited research into this area suggests that many managers and employers are not effectively skilled in managing staff of menopausal age and some women report that they have received criticism and even harassment directed at their menopause-related sick leave. There are moves to improve this situation. In the recent Diversity Council Australia and Australian Human Rights Commission report entitled *Older Women Matter: Harnessing the Talents of Australia's Older Female Workforce*, the authors examined the specific experiences of women aged over forty-five in employment. They present an organisational framework that proposes to increase women's workforce contributions and improve working conditions for women. Notional solutions to increase support of women in the menopause transition include education, environmental modification and changes to workplace culture.

Case study: Management tale

For all the management training that I went through and advice I had received, nothing quite prepared me for the experience of managing a team member suffering from chronic health issues related to menopause.

As a man, my understanding of menopause was basic (at best) and steeped in myths and assumptions. Much like my understanding of the menstrual cycle, I knew of it, understood it generally wasn't a very nice experience for women to go through and certainly was keen to avoid talking about it directly due to my overall ignorance on the subject.

My team member first brought menopause to light after a string of medical appointments she needed to attend that meant she would come in late or leave early. As a manager and as a business we have always supported flexible working hours and locations so this was well within reason. Prompted by a question as to what support she needed at this time in light of the medical appointments, it was explained to me that she was going through the change that women of her age do and that this had an impact on her health.

The use of the term 'the change' framed it in a way that led me to assume this was a short-term thing that would run its course. The topic of her health was addressed at our regular one to one catch-ups when needed as we continued to have open, albeit surface-level, dialogue. In the weeks that followed, the health issues continued with a range of stomach-aches and pains, through to headaches and nausea, so too did medical appointments. I did seek advice at that stage from our local HR team, who generally talked around menopause with statements like it affects women differently.

It was also around this time that my team member started discussing medication that was being prescribed to address her health issues. Again, the language and tone of the conversations with both HR and the team member implied a simplicity to the issue that would lead to a simple resolution. It was when the team member moved onto medication that I saw the biggest impact not just on her health but her overall wellbeing. Aside from migraines, aches and pains, what was most striking was her chronic and drastic mood swings. The highs were few and far between, with her mood and general demeanour moving into unpredictable and worryingly depressive tendencies. This would manifest itself as her being very demotivated, disengaged, negative and aggressive. Probably the worst incident was when she disclosed to another team member that she didn't know what she was living for any more.

The advice from our HR team didn't really empower me to try to help the team member outside of advising of the employee assistance program and advising on leave and flexible working options. This was hugely uncharted territory for me, and outside of asking what can we do to support her from a work perspective, I felt incredibly helpless and concerned for her.

I shared my concerns for her health and wellbeing with her on a number of occasions, directly asking if she was OK and what support could we as an organisation provide to her. The response was usually the same – 'Thanks, I'm working through some stuff at the moment, which is very hard, and appreciate the support.'

I started to question, shamefully, whether my supportive nature was being taken advantage of or not, and decided to do some basic reading into the menopause – and yes Wikipedia was the starting point. The research I did made me realise there wasn't going to be a quick resolution to her symptoms and acknowledge that the work solution was about how work could support the management of her symptoms. This changed the tone and structure of our conversations moving forwards and certainly made me more confident in talking to her about what she was going through.

Having seen first-hand the impact menopause can have on a woman's health, I wish I had known what I know now earlier on; I certainly would have been more explicit in our discussions rather than sheepishly dancing around the issue.

Self-care: Succeed at work

For managers and employers there are several ways that menopausal women can be supported when dealing with common symptoms. These steps include:

- **Knowledge and respect.** Get informed. Understanding menopause and knowing that it is a healthy, normal but long process is crucial. Compassion and respect are also essential. Recognising that menopause is a consequence of women's fertility, and acknowledging that symptoms exist because of that, may help.

- **Encourage conversation.** The fact that fifty-odd per cent of the population go through menopause, which is a sign of health, makes it common and not a taboo subject. It is normal and natural. Ensure staff understand how menopause can affect work and discuss what adjustments can be made and what support is available.

- **Control over temperature.** Offering control over ambient temperature such as windows that open, installation of fans, or simply placing work desks by windows to get breezes can help women manage hot flushes. Temperature control with reverse-cycle air-conditioning units for large spaces are not helpful – some people freeze, while others cook. Desk fans and more localised options are more suitable. Hot desking and open plan offices do not support women's ability to manage symptoms.

- **Flexibility.** Flexible work hours that allow for menopause-related sick leave and the need for medical appointments. Quiet respite opportunities such as encouraging staff to take lunch breaks away from the office, having stand and stretch breaks during long meetings, conferences or other business occasions. Providing seating options for retail workers if required, and making sure shift workers take leave and breaks as needed, even if that inconveniences the team. Cultivating a culture where self-care is important and holidays and annual leave are to be taken regularly.

- **Dress code and/or uniform options.** Uniforms that include layers are helpful, such as cardigans and jackets, as well as removing tight-fitting belts and avoiding tight-waisted clothes. Dresses, for example, are better than shirts tucked in and belted, and compulsory neck scarves or high-necked garments can be diabolical for hot flushes. Consider the dress code with a woman's comfort in mind, as that will improve her work productivity.

- **Cold water on tap.** Providing ready access to cold water and/or accessible bathrooms are two very practical strategies.

Summary: Nurturing relationships and celebrating roles

Positive and satisfactory relationships and roles improve physical and mental health and support optimal quality of life. Menopause and midlife may feature changes in our significant relationships, associated roles, interests and priorities in life, but because they are so important to our wellbeing it is important that we get them right so we can get maximal enjoyment from the next stage of life.

- **Focus on the good.** Find the good in all your chosen relationships and recognise the strengths of the people you surround yourself with. Each relationship is unique, and diversity in our relationships provides greater health and wellbeing benefits. Focusing on the good within yourself is crucial too.
- **Fleece the negative.** With age we become more aware of how time is precious. Consider spending your time in ways that energise, validate and support you and remove the things that don't. This may mean a change in relationships and friendships that are energy draining rather than life enhancing. Or it could mean surrendering roles and responsibilities that are no longer fulfilling or have exceeded their original purpose.
- **Love and appreciate.** Love generously and spend time with people who are important to you. Connect and be compassionate rather than comparing or competing.

Appreciate the ones you love. When things are changing, it can be difficult to keep this in mind if you focus instead on confronting difference. Appreciate and celebrate what remains important and constant.

- **Engage and achieve.** The shift from reproductive function provides the opportunity to take on new roles and relationships or to re-engage with previous roles and activities. Expand your life outwards rather than contract it inwards. Set new goals for yourself and start to accomplish them. Now is the time to start actioning the list of things you want to do and to stop delaying or postponing them. How do you want to spend your last thirty summers?

- **Find meaning and purpose.** Menopause is an ideal time for women to recalibrate their lives, as they are free from cycling hormones – their bodies, brains, emotions and behaviour are different. Identify what gives you a sense of meaning and purpose. What makes your soul sing? What is your legacy going to be? What do you want to create, accomplish, bequeath, love? Find what is important, then prioritise and action it in your life.

PART 6

MENOPAUSE MANAGEMENT MAP

Menopause is a natural rite of passage, not a biological failure. It is a process we can actively manage in order to reduce discomfort as well as invest in our health and wellbeing into our future. Menopause does not require medical treatment per se, as it is not a disease and there is no cure. Any conceptualisation of menopause as a hormone deficit is inappropriate, as your body is pre-programmed to decrease hormones and adjust. If menopause were characterised as a hormone deficiency, then puberty would be viewed as a hormone excess, rather than them being the bookends to our reproductive years.

It is important to keep this in mind, as it is easy to be swept up in the over-medicalisation of menopause rather than accepting it as natural and applying lifestyle and mindstyle strategies for symptom management. There is an important differentiation between symptom management and the treatment of hormone decline. I know of an older woman who has been taking hormone replacement for over fifteen years and now feels dependent upon them and fears menopause, so she wants to take hormones for the rest of her life. For the majority intervention provides a temporary reprieve, as the primary purpose of management or intervention is to relieve the frequency and intensity of symptoms that cause discomfort and reduce quality of life. The second objective of intervention is to reduce health risks and prevent chronic medical conditions associated with menopause and increasing age, such as cardiovascular disease and osteoporosis.

Your first option with menopause is to do nothing, and about one third of women do this and require no intervention. Along with their rejection of the medicalisation of this female process, women also often cite the competing and confusing claims regarding products and product harms as a reason for this decision. Allowing menopause to proceed naturally and using lifestyle and mindstyle strategies to enhance health and reduce symptoms is very effective for many women.

Being open to seeing how the menopause transition unfolds, rather than perhaps pre-emptively thinking it will be challenging and commencing treatment, is helpful to minimise unnecessary treatment. I have heard women say that as soon as they detect symptoms they will commence HT (hormone therapy), but with almost half of women not experiencing significant symptoms that might not be sensible, especially given the adverse risks associated with taking hormones. However, it is also important to remain open to the possibility that assistance or management strategies may be necessary to maintain quality of life.

Half of all women in menopause find that management of their symptoms is necessary. There are plenty of treatment options available and the difficult thing is negotiating all the information, claims and counterclaims and risks associated with supplements, nutraceuticals, hormone therapy and alternative health practices. Previously the only option was hormone replacement treatment. Now there are multiple offerings, including a raft of new non-hormonal pharmacological treatments developed along with new bio-identical hormones, complementary offerings and alternative herbal and other remedies. Many have no supporting evidence to back up their claims. However, a recent survey of women found that over half were using complementary medicines and that many women have swung back to HT.

I suggest taking a bigger step back and seeing the transition as one aspect of your global health and psychological wellbeing.

Consider your health, lifestyle, mindstyle, relationships, roles and environment, as well as your inner self, dreams and goals. Make necessary changes in a holistic manner that will ultimately serve you better than simply adopting management or treatment options. A big-picture view will allow you to see causal contributing factors that you can address. For example, there is little point in taking hormones or sleeping tablets to address sleep disturbance if the real culprit is drinking coffee in the afternoon.

Because there are many options, it is vital to consider symptoms, issues and choices so that you can tailor management to your individual needs. Many menopause symptoms are temporary, so a regular review of your status and management may be necessary as menopause progresses. There are a multitude of options and we may require multiple forms of management depending on what symptoms are causing the greatest impact on our wellbeing. The constant focus of intervention must be to reduce the negative impact and disruption to your quality of life as well as prevent risk and minimise harm.

Starting your management plan

Be prepared. As peri-menopause usually starts when children are in school, as careers are settling, and as age-related health changes start, this is a crucial time to take stock and improve your general health. For most women changes in menses start to occur when they are in their forties, and for some women their thirties. With that in mind perhaps observe your cycle and become familiar with its idiosyncrasies so that you can detect any changes. When you become aware of any changes make a note of them and decide if they are an issue or problem for you at the time. Consider your next steps.

The first appointment is most likely to be with your general practitioner or other health professional and the immediate question will be whether you are experiencing peri-menopause.

Changes to menses do not necessarily mean you are in the menopause transition. A differential diagnosis is necessary to rule out other hormone disturbances or other medical and health issues such as stress or rapid weight change.

To make that first appointment most effective, prepare answers to these questions, which you will most likely be asked by the health practitioner: When was your last period? What are your symptoms – type, frequency, intensity? What are you doing to alleviate your symptoms? What makes them worse? What appears to reduce the severity and/or frequency of them? What is your general health history? Any family medical issues? Your knowledge about yourself is important.

You may have questions too. Write them down so you remember them and make notes of the answers or record the session. Simple or obvious considerations include what tests are necessary (for example, blood tests or ovarian ultrasound); symptom management options; websites or helpful information sources; and health maintenance. Please get the practitioner to consider your entire medical history and any other medical health issues, disease risks and family history such as cardiovascular disease, diabetes, obesity and osteoporosis.

Quick tips: Planning your appointment

- **Review your general health**. Conduct an honest review of your general health and lifestyle to identify what is harming or enhancing your health and write it down to share with your health practitioner.
- **Record your symptoms**. Make a list of your symptoms, their frequency and intensity. For example, note down the number of hot flushes you experience each day or week and note how severe they are on a one to five scale. Note if there are any factors that impact them.

- **Document everything**. List all medications, and any herbs, vitamin supplements and nutraceuticals you take and include how much and how often.
- **Write your questions down**. There will be a lot to discuss so list your questions and work through them with the doctor. Take a notepad or record the session so you don't forget the answers.
- **Identify your support team**. Think of the supportive people in your life and recruit their support as necessary – a problem shared is a problem halved. It may also be helpful to take a support person with you to appointments, so you can discuss and brainstorm afterwards.

Healthy lifestyle

Maintaining a healthy foundation not only reduces disease risk and facilitates recovery, it supports daily function and quality of life. Our overall health is the product of both our physical body and our state of mind (described below in Positive mindstyle, see pages 240–4). A healthy lifestyle is relatively widely understood in terms of diet, sleep, exercise, low substance use and managing medical issues. The links between the body and mind hold true across our entire lifespan, and menopause is no different. Now is a great time to evaluate your lifestyle, and mindstyle, because the hormonal changes directly impact the body, brain and mind, and your mind impacts upon your brain and body.

Lifestyle is largely under your control and will make a big difference to your experience of the menopause transition. Consider your level of physical fitness, muscle strength, fat mass, diet, sleep, mental health and substance use.

List the areas of your lifestyle you think are not helpful to you and your menopause transition. Identify those that are a priority for you to address based on your values and what is important. List all your menopause symptoms and ask yourself, Are any linked to lifestyle habits? Then rate how much of a problem each symptom is for you. This is more important than simply listing the frequency or intensity of symptoms: it is possible to have a menopause symptom that is not a problem and that doesn't bother you, so don't treat it. Think of a woman with lower libido and vaginal dryness who, with her partner, decided the change to their sexual intimacy was not an issue as they were so invested in their emotional intimacy and other areas of their relationship.

Investigate the best and most helpful lifestyle changes you can make and perhaps discuss them with your treating health professional, partner and/or close supportive friends, and then determine how to best make necessary changes. Visualise the change and consider how the change will improve your quality of life, especially if it involves a beloved or deeply ingrained habit or addiction – even say to yourself, 'When I do X I will feel Y,' as this confirms your intention and will help you stay motivated. A subtraction has been found easier to manage than making an addition. What lifestyle habits undermine your current level of health and wellbeing? Consider things such as smoking cigarettes, drinking too much alcohol, eating discretionary foods daily. Adopting new lifestyle habits that enhance health, such as regular physical exercise and practising optimism, takes planning and time as well as commitment. Be patient and kind with yourself while you make changes as it is hard to alter habits.

You may find that your symptoms improve immediately, and the transition becomes easier to manage. Some changes may take longer to yield results, so maintain motivation by reaffirming that you are investing in yourself and your future. Know that your improved health will support you to thrive in the next stage of your life. It may also reduce your need to introduce medications or alternative options into your body, with their side effects and changes to the natural process.

Investigate which changes work for you by conducting your own experiment. Start by getting your baseline, which means rating the symptom frequency and/or intensity for a week before you make any changes, and then monitor the differences for a month. It is necessary to sustain the change for four weeks, as your body will take some time to adjust. One change with a big impact may be all you need to do during the transition. For example, alcohol is an easy and obvious target because it has profound effects on hormones, cancer risk, sleep disturbance, weight gain, energy levels, hot flushes and more. Try stopping or reducing your alcohol intake for a month and see if your night flushes reduce in frequency and/or if sleep disturbance improves and monitor for any other changes.

Another easy lifestyle target to change which has a big positive impact is sleep. Many people take products to help with sleep but have poor sleep hygiene practices, such as drinking coffee late in the afternoon, drinking alcohol each night, watching television in bed, and having no regular bedtime routine or sleep time. Consequently, they take medications or other products to help with sleep that leave them groggy and slow in the morning, whereas sleep issues may be entirely manageable through lifestyle. Unlike treatments, a healthy lifestyle does not have negative side effects.

Your health status and lifestyle habits as you enter menopause and midlife significantly determine your health and quality of life in late life. Live and age successfully, which the World Health Organization terms active aging, and which involves an active process of ongoing participation in social, economic, cultural, spiritual and civic affairs, along with being physically active, independent and optimally healthy.

Aging as a normal process can be healthy or can be characterised by chronic disease. With increasing medical technology, we can measure the aging process – natural and diseased. We can then compare a person's chronological age and normal aging processes with their physiological age and changes due to lifestyle and disease. This is important as most of today's non-communicable diseases are lifestyle based, caused by behaviours such as eating an unhealthy diet, smoking, drinking excessive alcohol and not engaging in physical exercise. These lifestyle patterns are linked to type II diabetes, cardiovascular disease, stroke, some cancers and dementia, as well as contributing to disabilities. An Australian woman today whose average lifespan is projected to be about eighty-four years is only likely to enjoy good health and independence for the first sixty-four years and then to live with some form of health issue or disability for the remainder. But it does not have to be the case.

The clear message from current medical research is that your lifestyle in midlife, from the amount of exercise you engage in to how much muscle mass you have, along with the nutritional value of your diet, and your attitude and mental health, fundamentally impact upon your ability to live well in your later years. The best investments you can make for your late life are not just financial ones but health ones. Start with the high-return investments of being a healthy weight with regular exercise and a good level of fitness. Fuel yourself with highly nutritious healthy food and prioritise sleep to allow restoration and repair, and then limit the health taxes of excessive alcohol, cigarettes, recreational drugs and stress.

Diet and menopause

A healthy diet provides all the essential nutrients, energy and protein we require for optimal health, which includes hormone production and regulation as well as fuelling the hungriest organ of the body – the brain. As many as ninety-five per cent of adults do not follow the daily dietary recommendation for vegetable consumption. Our dietary requirements vary depending upon our energy expenditure, genetic make-up, health and age. During menopause when our hormone levels are changing we are especially sensitive to hormone dysfunction from an unhealthy diet, with the results being fatigue, weight gain, stress, low mood, increased hot flushes, disturbed sleep and increased disease risk.

As we age we also need to be more vigilant about what we eat, as metabolism can change and we absorb fewer of the nutrients in our food and our taste sensitivity decreases. We need to eat more high-quality nutritious foods and fewer empty carbohydrates, and increase the flavour of our food without increasing salt, sugar and fat by using herbs and spices and other flavourful ingredients.

The recommendation is to follow a healthy diet as a priority and add in supplements etc if necessary. Plan your meals so you always have a healthy and diverse food intake, with low saturated fat and plenty of proteins from eggs, chicken and fish along with complex carbohydrates such as brown rice, legumes, pulses, whole grains, and a wide variety of vegetables and one to two serves of fruit. When you have a healthy and nutritious eating pattern it is possible to add sometimes foods – dessert, cakes, snacks, chocolate or other treats.

If that diet is not sufficient in providing your required dietary needs due to absorption issues or medical concerns, then add supplements as recommended. You may need calcium, iron or vitamin D, as women of increasing age often require supplements even with a healthy diet. Always check with your health provider, though, as some supplements and nutraceuticals negatively interact with medications or can cause serious health issues if taken in excess where there is no need.

In terms of diet and menopause there is a smorgasbord of dietary suggestions and even specific diet protocols. However, when reviewed by medical research teams very few of the diet claims are supported by scientific research. One area of consensus is that women during the menopause transition, and as they continue to age, need to monitor their intake of calcium and iron, as these are often low in their food intake. Your iron and calcium levels can be checked via a blood test if you have concerns and should only be supplemented following medical advice. Natural sources of calcium are found in dairy products, fish with bones such as sardines and canned salmon, broccoli, parsley and legumes, while iron is best obtained from eating red meat.

Diet does impact hot flushes, and not just in terms of what you eat but also how often you eat. A fall in blood glucose levels, which happens between meals or after high sugar intake, is linked to an increase in hot flushes. Eating meals reduces the frequency of hot flushes, so if you are a person who has irregular meals or skips them entirely rethink your eating patterns. Breakfast is important to stabilise blood glucose levels for the entire day and so is eating every four to five hours, so keep to a routine of regular meals. Studies examining blood glucose levels and skin heat conduction indicate that after eating, women can enjoy on average ninety minutes without hot flushes. In contrast, the longer time between meals increased flushes. Eating regularly and having a small snack in between meals if necessary to keep blood glucose stable could make a huge difference in the number of flushes.

Science bite: Glucose and flushes

Blood glucose levels and hot flushes are believed to be linked because the brain requires a continuous glucose supply to function, with delivery via the bloodstream. Glucose levels are constantly being regulated and controlled by the brain, blood glucose levels and the neurovascular system. Oestrogen plays a role in this system by improving the amount and transportation of available glucose

---

when demand increases. According to the glucose model of hot flushes there is less oestrogen to help regulate the system and the hot flush is an over-compensating response when glucose levels are low, so that the blood vessels dilate to increase glucose and oxygen flow to meet the brain's glucose needs. In simple terms your body gets hot because blood vessels have expanded to get glucose upstairs to your brain in a hurry.

There is plenty of evidence that certain foods increase hot flushes and night sweats. The chief offenders are alcohol, caffeine, excess sugar, meat products and spicy food like garlic, ginger and chilli, and hot drinks which increase your temperature. They all increase flushes and sweats by different pathways – excess sugar impacts glucose and insulin levels, caffeine acts as a stimulant that excites the cardiovascular and sympathetic nervous systems, and meat and dairy trigger inflammatory processes which can increase adrenaline and the sympathetic nervous system. Another food to avoid or reduce is carbonated soft drinks, which may deplete the body of calcium and therefore increase the risk of bone loss and osteoporosis.

There are also foods with specific compounds that are thought to decrease hot flushes, but the evidence remains controversial. Probably the most common foods are those that contain phytoestrogens, such as soy, alfalfa, red clover and flaxseeds. Phytoestrogens appear to reduce the frequency of hot flushes, as they have oestrogen-like properties. Other helpful foods are those high in omega-3 fatty acids, such as oily fish, and they also help manage cholesterol and therefore reduce cardiovascular disease risk. Antioxidants, especially vitamins C and E from dark-coloured vegetables and fruits, are good for reducing inflammation, which helps hormone production and regulation.

Eating healthy foods in the right quantities has no negative side effects and your health will improve even if hot flushes do not change. Additionally, many of the helpful foods have additional benefits to health, such as reducing disease risks for cancer and cardiovascular disease and improving gut health. None of the food sources of phytoestrogens and antioxidants or with anti-inflammatory properties need to be exotic, expensive or imported, or require a specific product or diet to be obtained: your local fresh produce shop will have them all.

The other important thing to consider is your level of hydration. Drink plenty of water every day and increase your intake in hot weather and with exercise. Good hydration supports all bodily processes including hormone production and regulation. Often, we think we are hungry when we are thirsty, so being hydrated is important for appetite regulation as well as helping with waste management and metabolism.

Once you have established foundational healthy habits – strategies and options provided at the end of each section of the book – and you are still experiencing symptoms and discomfort, consider other management and treatment options.

Positive mindstyle

Mindstyle is not something most people are familiar with or understand. Essentially mindstyle means how we think, including our beliefs, self-talk and attitude. A healthy mindstyle involves self-acceptance, resilience, good stress management, a positive outlook, enjoying positive emotional experiences, a sense of contentment, and meaning and purpose. Optimistic, hopeful and positive thoughts bring a feeling of contentment and calmness, as well as significantly boosting mental and physical health. We can choose to cultivate a positive mindstyle in the same way we can practice a healthy lifestyle.

Our mindstyle is very important as we arrive at menopause in midlife and are increasingly aware we are aging. Often our thoughts about menopause and aging are intertwined and not always in a helpful way. Women undergo physical, cognitive and psychological changes associated with increasing life years and changes due to menopause. It can be difficult to separate them out medically and it can be complicated for women as individuals to understand the role of each and balance the changes of both. We get wrinkles with increasing age, and we get wrinkles from loss of oestrogen in menopause. Wrinkles express our life story. A truism that is often taken for granted is that if we were not alive we wouldn't get wrinkles. At some level it is necessary to appreciate and be thankful for the life experiences one has had and for the opportunity to have more.

As one of my clients stated, think that every day above ground is a blessing. In previous generations menopause signalled imminent death. A woman born in 1930 lived on average only sixty-one years. They were lucky to get through to post-menopause. Today, by contrast, the female lifespan stretches to over eighty years. The menopause transition occurs in midlife not late life, with most women having at least another twenty years in which to continue to bloom. One of my friends turning fifty stated, we have another thirty summers. What is important is to make those years good ones.

While other cultures view older age as the stage of maturity and wisdom, in Western societies, becoming an older woman has not been valued. The central issue is the continuing association of female beauty and attractiveness with sex and youth. Attitudes in society are beginning to shift, albeit slowly, but the first place to start is actually how we relate to ourselves. We are all physically aging at the same rate – one moment at a time – regardless of how old we are. Enjoy getting older: it is a privilege. It also means you have had more time on the planet, more time to love and be loved, more time to journey. If you worry about the notion of becoming 'invisible', or no longer attractive, change your mindset. Women in midlife today are becoming increasingly visible and assertive. They have been educated and have rich experiences under their belt and more goals and dreams ahead of them. That said, being sexually 'invisible' can be very liberating. You do not need to worry what others think and you no longer need external approval. Rather, invest in developing your own style and feeling attractive in your own eyes and focus your energy on your personal priorities. Celebrate a new confident you. Increasing age makes us more unique. Value your uniqueness: it is more attractive than youthfulness.

Age well – it is a mindset. Everything you previously thought about midlife and aging is likely to be wrong. Forget the stereotypes. Friendships change, they become deeper and more intimate as we tend to value quality over quantity with age. As a result, adults in midlife report less loneliness, more supportive friendships, less conflict and better marriages than younger adults. We also become more content with age, and this feeling of satisfaction increases steadily from midlife well into late life. The idea that people become sadder or more depressed with age also doesn't hold true, as with age we focus more on the positives and we find meaning and satisfaction more often than not. Clarify your thoughts on aging, your values and goals, and consider how you want your midlife and late life to unfold.

Midlife is a major transition stage in adult development where our past experiences and future expectations get cross referenced, we reconcile pains and joys and we develop new dreams and plans to move forwards. Menopause is a great signpost in life to improve your psychological wellbeing and empower your future.

Western medicine does not adequately integrate the psychological stages of life with the physical processes of living and health. Although mental processes and psychological tensions transmit into physiological experiences, which can affect health and disease risks, western medicine tends to separate these elements out. Menopause is similarly not seen as a stage of psychological growth. In contrast, eastern medicine does integrate the body, brain and energy/soul and has a framework that might be helpful. They perceive menopause as the movement of creative life forces from the uterus and other sexual organs to the heart. What makes your heart or soul sing?

Psychologists have investigated midlife and recognise specific important tasks in our development. Erik Erickson described midlife as the seventh stage in human maturation and recognised it as an important time for establishing balance between generativity versus stagnation. The term generativity refers to energy to care for others, be creative and accomplish things. A time to 'make your mark' and realise your strengths and unique offerings. The opposing force is termed stagnation and describes the failure to find a way to contribute, a lack of meaning and purpose, a sense of being uninvolved or disconnected. Menopause provides women with freedom from sexual reproduction and thereby supports growth and expansion.

Carl Jung described midlife in a similar vein as a time crucial for self-realisation, when we have a dawning understanding of ourselves and our capacity to flourish while confronting our weaknesses ('one's shadow'). It is seen as a time when we begin to accept ourselves and recognise our identities and authentic selves and understand that we will not live forever. This creates momentum to achieve and grow. One task now is to look outwards, to optimistically and positively open oneself up to opportunities and new experiences.

What are your dreams? How will you be creative and enjoy generativity and self-realisation versus stagnation? What interests do you want to pursue? What goals are there yet to achieve and roles yet to be realised? How do you want to live every season as if it is summer?

The other task is to know, accept and respect oneself. By the time women reach menopause and midlife, most have mastered love for others (their parents, partners, friends and children) so now is a good time to focus love upon themselves. The relationship we have with ourselves is the most important one we have. Bring your attitude, psychological frame of mind and physical health together. Become intimate with yourself – know your heart, mind, body and spirit. Celebrate yourself. Now is the time to truly integrate those aspects of yourself and to live in a way that is true to your genuine self, so you blossom.

Supplements, nutraceuticals and botanicals

Aside from a healthy normal diet there are increasing numbers of dietary supplements, nutraceuticals, herbal remedies and other botanicals being marketed to improve health. It is estimated that up to seventy per cent of adults take some form of supplement daily and the industry is worth billions of dollars. Due to the reporting of adverse risks associated with pharmacological treatments, more people are turning to supplements and nutraceuticals. However, many have negative side effects that need to be considered along with their benefits.

In well-nourished adults who eat a healthy diet and who do not have medical and/or absorption issues, there is no evidence that dietary supplements provide health benefits and some products can in fact cause significant toxicity. They can also interact with medications and other supplements. They may be beneficial but not because of the active agents in them. Recent understanding suggests that up to half or more of the benefit from interventions (of any form) may be due to the powerful 'placebo' effect, meaning the positive expectation of benefit *causes* benefit, due in whole or part to changes in brain chemistry which signal to the body that positive effects are being experienced.

There are many products that purport to relieve menopause by reducing the severity and frequency of symptoms. Many are described as natural and are derived from plant sources, with the implication that they are good for you and won't be harmful. This is not necessarily true – arsenic, for example, is a natural substance and it is potentially lethal. Not every health product, even those purporting to be natural, is beneficial, and some have serious adverse effects.

The evidence that these natural remedies are beneficial is limited and, worse, there is an absence of evidence of their potential harms because they are not investigated. This is because there is no government regulation of supplements as there is of food products and pharmaceuticals. Consider the implications of this for a second: there is no control over the type of ingredients, the quality and amount of the ingredients, nor is there investigation into the benefits or harms of the product. There is also no significant control over the active compounds, dose and duration of use. The lack of regulation introduces multiple risks to the consumer. The other issue is that often the practitioners selling you these products get a direct profit or kickback from the sale.

Common symptoms of adverse reactions to supplements, nutraceuticals and botanicals range from nausea, fatigue and headache to more severe toxicity, liver damage, oxidative stress and alterations to subtle physiological process such as bile acid homeostasis and mitochondrial dysfunction, whereby cells can't process energy and potentially die.

Herbs, roots and other plant derivatives have been used by humans for aeons as 'medical' treatments and can be considered as precursors to many of the pharmacological treatments we have today. It is natural and logical to consider them when trying to improve overall health and to remedy medical conditions, as supplements and as treatments respectively. Like pharmaceuticals, supplements and nutraceuticals can also have adverse effects and cause toxicity.

The most widely consumed supplements are those derived from fruits, vegetables and herbs and are often high in anti-inflammatory and/or antioxidant properties, which are very beneficial to us. I suggest eating foods high in those properties rather than the supplement form, as many foods have synergistic properties that increase the benefits of other foods and often have more than one single benefit. For example, you could take an anti-inflammatory tablet or eat foods high in flavonoids such as dark chocolate. Eating small amounts of dark chocolate also helps maintain vascular tone and insulin sensitivity and stimulates improved mood, so the additional benefits of a piece of chocolate are heart health, brain health and joy.

There are many different products available, so what is documented here is not an exhaustive list but, rather, some suggestions of products that are currently being marketed for menopause symptom relief, particularly hot flushes. My commitment is to provide information, so you can make the best choices for yourself, and only to report on those areas where there is some level of scientific evidence. There are many other supplements and nutraceuticals to manage more general symptoms, such as poor sleep, muscle tension and fatigue. One is magnesium, which is an essential mineral for optimal health and commonly used to assist sleep and as a muscle relaxant – this use is supported by research.

However, the cautions given above are relevant to all products. Additionally, most people don't report using them to their primary medical practitioners and risk the negative interactive consequences of these type of treatments with prescribed medications, so always discuss everything with your doctor.

Science bite: Phytoestrogens

Phytoestrogens occur naturally in certain foods. There are two main types of phytoestrogens — isoflavones and lignans. Isoflavones are found in soybeans, lentils, chickpeas and other legumes, and lignans occur in flaxseed, whole grains and some fruits and vegetables. Phytoestrogens have a similar molecular structure to oestradiol and can bond to oestrogen receptors in the body, albeit weakly, and therefore have weak oestrogen-like effects and may help reduce the number of hot flushes. The Asian diet includes more phytoestrogen-rich foods and studies suggest that Asian women have fewer vasomotor symptoms than American women, although other studies suggest that they report symptoms less rather than experience them less.

Phytoestrogens

Phytoestrogens (plant oestrogens) are found in certain foods and impact female reproductive hormones and are now increasingly being packaged as hormone supplements or nutraceuticals for women in the menopause transition. Surveys suggest that approximately forty per cent of American women use soy products, and some go as far as to use isoflavone extracts and purified isoflavones such as genistein, although, like all oestrogen-increasing treatment there is the suggestion that high doses are likely to increase the risks of oestrogen-sensitive cancers just as medical hormone treatments do. The benefit of phytoestrogens such as isoflavones varies depending upon the oestrogen receptor they bind to, how much oestrogen is already in the body, and even the type of gut bacteria you have with which to metabolise it in the first place. It is suggested that only thirty per cent of women will benefit, and under rigorous examination there was no evidence that phytoestrogen supplements effectively reduce the frequency or severity of hot flushes and night sweats in women compared to a placebo. It also needs to be noted that in clinical trials adverse side effects following prescribed phytoestrogen intake have been reported. Additionally, the longer-term adverse effects of phytoestrogen use on heart diseases, breast cancer and stroke remain unknown.

Black cohosh

The herb black cohosh has been used in menopause to treat hot flashes, sweats, mood changes and other symptoms. However, it was traditionally used by Native American to treat menstrual issues and its application to menopause has occurred without studies to support its use. Because of its apparent effects black cohosh has undergone formal investigation. A review of sixteen clinical trials involving over two thousand women found no evidence to support its use to treat menopause. It was found that black cohosh did not act like oestrogen, which was positive because that means it will not overstimulate oestrogen-sensitive tissue and therefore not increase breast and ovarian cancer risk. However, there is suggestion that it may cause liver damage. After an Australian study published its findings an American expert health panel (Therapeutic Goods Administration) made it statutory to include warning labels.

Red clover

Red clover is a plant that contains many edible parts, with the flowers used in supplements and the leaves in tea or in salads. Warning, high ingestion can cause bloating. Red clover is high in isoflavones, which you will recall are hormone-like molecules that are changed into phytoestrogens that lock onto oestrogen receptors. It is, therefore, used for hot flushes and breast tenderness in menopause. In human clinical studies there was no conclusive evidence that women who took red clover extract experienced any decrease in vasomotor symptoms. The risks of red clover are the same as all products that impact hormone function and oestrogen-sensitive tissue and cancer risk. Experts think it has also led to infertility in animals.

Ginseng

Ginseng has been used for an exceptionally long time in Chinese and Asian medicine as a healing and restorative tonic to treat multiple symptoms and conditions. It is derived from the plant root and the active ingredient is ginsenoside, which is believed to have properties that increase immune function. It has therefore been used in cancer treatment and there is suggestion that ginseng may also relieve mood and sleep disturbance symptoms linked to menopause, but there is no indication that it will impact hot flushes.

Evening primrose oil

Evening primrose oil is extracted from the plant's seed and contains essential omega-6 fatty acids, which decrease inflammation. It is a traditional medicinal plant for Native Americans and has been used for thousands of years. It has been used to relieve breast tenderness and premenstrual issues, and for skin conditions. It is now being repackaged for relief of hot flushes in menopause. However, the evidence for this benefit is not yet present.

Kava

Kava is a beverage extract drunk in the Pacific and is a psychoactive substance that affects mental and emotional processes in the brain. It is used for its relaxant properties – it reduces stress, anxiety and restlessness and has been packaged as a nutraceutical for treating sleep problems. There is evidence it may impact vasomotor function as it is a relaxant, and therefore may decrease hot flushes. However, it is, like other drugs such as alcohol, a burden on the body and is associated with increased risk of liver damage and liver disease.

St John's wort

St John's wort is a yellow-flowering shrub that is a curse for agriculture and animals but has been used for a long time to treat several nervous system conditions, such as low mood, lack of energy and stress. Because it appears to work on the stress response system, St John's wort is taken by some women to alleviate vasomotor symptoms. The evidence supporting its use for mood and stress is not matched by evidence for its use in menopause for hot flushes. It is better taken in the morning because known side effects are trouble sleeping, vivid dreams and restlessness. It can interfere with medication: for example, women taking tamoxifen must avoid it because St John's wort makes the medication ineffective.

Chinese herbal medicine

Due to increasing understanding and respect for non-western medical traditions and acceptance of acupuncture, more women are looking towards Chinese herbal medicine as an alternative therapy and to reduce adverse effects. However, the treatments may not be safe and often have not undergone the type of rigorous clinical trials that other forms of medical treatment must undergo. A review of the effectiveness and safety identified twenty-two studies involving almost three thousand women that compared Chinese herbal remedies to placebo treatment and found no difference in the severity of hot flushes or their frequency. When compared to HT, results were unclear. The adverse effects are different from those reported in HT studies, however, and include things like diarrhoea, gastric discomfort and unpleasant taste.

As with all the interventions described above, and those not yet known, please discuss your health and requirements with your treating doctor before taking any herbal or dietary supplements for menopausal symptoms. They are not regulated and have not undergone the same quality of production and manufacturing or the same level of research scrutiny that pharmacological medications have undergone. Some can be dangerous or interact with other medications you may be taking, putting your health at risk.

Self-care: Monitor 'natural' options

- **Use with caution**. Just because it is natural does not mean it does not have risks. Investigate the risks. Monitor quality (that is, purity, percentage, dose of the active agent) and production (for example, sterility, other ingredients) and know what other non-active ingredients are in the product.
- **Inform your doctor**. Always inform your medical doctor and all other health practitioners of all supplements, botanicals and nutraceuticals you take in order to minimise drug interactions and toxicity. Be sure to also stop all types of treatments at least two weeks before you have planned surgery.
- **Monitor your use**. Consider what benefit you want or what symptoms you are treating and rate the experience. Write down the start date you begin to use the product and reassess the symptom/s daily for a month: is there any change or side effects or other changes? For example, if you are considering taking black cohosh for hot flushes, note how many flushes you have per day and how intense they are before you start, and then continue to monitor frequency and intensity for a month while taking it.

Medical options

Menopause is not a medical condition but there are medical treatments that may alleviate symptoms, and for the minority of women who really suffer with their menopause symptoms these treatments are a godsend. The primary medical or pharmacological treatment for menopause is to increase hormone levels to relieve hot flushes. Other medical options include low doses of antidepressants and psychotropic medications, along with medication to prevent osteoporosis and manage other disease risks associated with increasing age.

All medications have adverse side effects and, as with nutraceuticals and alternative treatments, there is a significant placebo effect. It is important to talk over medication and side effects with your treating doctor and I also suggest getting a second opinion or consulting a specialist, so you can understand all your options and consider all risks and benefits. You will also need to review your treatment regimen alongside any other forms of management, medications and lifestyle and mindstyle strategies.

Case study: Court order

At fifty-two my periods had been intermittent for the previous year, with maybe one very heavy one and then nothing for a couple of months. I had never had any menstrual problems at all, aside from a little cramping on day one, and really couldn't understand what the fuss was all about even when I was a teenager.

I'd been married for fifteen years at this stage and had a previous live-in relationship, but have no children. I really wanted a child, but both of my partners had children from previous relationships and neither would have more.

I work as a legal professional and was living and working in a regional part of Australia. I lived in a regional city and was required to travel to work in other cities and towns in the area. Three weeks in four I was away from home from Monday morning to Friday night. My husband stayed in our capital city home because of his work and we would see each other at the weekends, with him mostly visiting me.

I have a form of arthritis that is under control, but the medication I take means I need careful monitoring. I had a very good GP in my home city, but it was hard to see her because I usually wasn't in the city during the week.

My first, and only, menopausal symptom occurred when I was sitting in court one day. Suddenly I felt this heat form across in the middle of my chest. It then quickly travelled across my chest and up to my head, causing a deep flush to my naturally pale skin. It was incredibly distracting, as I was right in the middle of a case and trying to listen to the evidence. The heat left within a couple of minutes (it felt like half an hour) and I only became concerned when it happened again within an hour or so. The flushes (I do think the American word flash is probably more appropriate) just kept on happening. Over the following days a 'flushing pattern' established of every forty-five minutes, day and night.

While I found the flushing incredibly distracting at work, it was also embarrassing, with staff asking me whether I was all right because my face and chest quickly became so flushed. The real problem was when I was trying to sleep. I've always been a good sleeper and find it essential to my work performance and my general functioning. I have a tendency towards anxiety and I've found exercise and good-quality sleep are essential to keeping this under control.

The flushes were happening every forty-five minutes at night too. It was the middle of winter in a part of the country where the temperatures would usually be below zero in the middle of the night. I would get to sleep fine and then wake up forty-five minutes later boiling hot. So hot I would have to throw all the bedclothes off and open the French doors in my bedroom to let the cold in. I'd get back to sleep and then wake a little while later freezing cold and had to close the doors and pull the bedclothes back on. Getting back to sleep again I'd wake with another hot flush after forty-five minutes and it would start all over again. After two nights of this I was exhausted, and it was a real struggle to do my job. I put up with it for about a week.

Working away from my home, I went to a random (young male) GP (I'm sure my regular GP who was a mature-aged woman would have been much more sympathetic) who told me he wouldn't prescribe anything until I had blood tests done. He didn't believe it was a menopause problem because I had no associated sweating, I had no associated mood swings and I had no other menopausal symptoms.

He decided I had a thyroid problem. I found myself begging him to give me some HRT. It felt so undignified. Very reluctantly he agreed to give me only one month's worth of HRT until we got the blood test results back. Driving back to my hotel, I found a pharmacy and handed across my prescription. When the middle-aged pharmacist brought the medication to me he said, 'Has your doctor fully explained to you the dangers of this medication?'

I said, 'No, but I am really suffering and unable to sleep because of hot flushes and I can't do my job properly right now.' He said, 'Oh, surely it can't be that bad, it's a natural process.'

I lost it. I said, 'You listen to me. I feel like a heroin addict who has just got their hands on a prescription for fentanyl patches. I want the medicine now.'

He handed it over, but it infuriated me that someone who hadn't even examined me or taken my history and who wasn't a doctor felt he had the right to interfere in my situation. I have always been very careful with my health,

*am not overweight, have never smoked, have regular blood
tests and make sure my blood pressure and cholesterol are
regularly checked.*

*The average life expectancy for women in the US in
1900 (the only stats I could quickly find on the internet)
was forty-eight years, so maybe they didn't even live
long enough to get to menopause! Why does the natural-
process argument only ever seem to apply to female issues
like childbirth and menopause? I never seem to hear that
argument in relation to erectile dysfunction problems in
aging men!*

*Anyway, of course it wasn't a thyroid problem and my
regular GP was much more sympathetic to my situation.
Miraculously, the flushes disappeared completely within four
days of starting HRT. Talking to friends and colleagues who
had menopausal symptoms, I was really surprised at their
reluctance to use HRT. Instead, they were buying whacky
'natural remedies' off the internet containing goodness
knows what and not getting any proper relief.*

*After a year or so my GP put me on a lower dosage of
HRT, which also works fine. One thing that does annoy me
is that the government seems to only allow two repeats on
each prescription, so I am regularly at the GP to get another
script. When I couldn't see my regular GP, another young
male GP told me I had to get off it immediately because of
the health risks. I discussed it with my regular GP on my
next visit and she said to give it a try, but I should remember
that some of the publicised research was now proven to be
unreliable and that the Queen Mother was on HRT until the
day she died [at age 101].*

*I did try to come off HRT last year, when I was fifty-six,
but the flushes were still there, although at reduced severity
and at increased intervals. Thank God for HRT!!!*

Hormone therapy

Hormone therapy (HT) remains a controversial treatment option. Some people get hot under the collar in the debate and I don't mean with a hot flush. Being passionate about a form of treatment is not always helpful, as high emotions tend to undermine thoughtful decision making and reduce capacity to respect different choices. The best suggestion is to remember that each of us has expert self-knowledge and is capable of making our own personal choices for our own reasons and priorities.

We all make our own hormones and if we are healthy and have a nutritious diet we can make what the body requires, as it has a very complex and well-designed feedback regulation system. The hormones we make ourselves are called endogenous hormones and the ones prescribed are called exogenous hormones.

There are plenty of times in a woman's reproductive lifespan that she may take exogenous hormonal treatments such as birth control (the contraceptive pill) and as treatment for endometriosis, infertility, dysfunctional uterine bleeding and menopause. However, just be aware that the World Health Organization states *all* exogenous hormones increase cancer risk, be it contraception or hormone therapy. Research continues to confirm that the longer hormones are taken, the greater the risks.

The first generation of hormone treatments for menopause generally consisted of equine oestrogen (from female horse pee) and medroxyprogesterone. The controversy regarding hormone replacement treatment for menopause stems from early research that suggested that HRT had serious health risks. There have been two exceedingly large studies, one in the USA called the Women's Health Initiative (WHI) and the other in the UK called the Million Women Study (MWS). These studies demonstrated that hormone therapy, replacing human molecular substances with inexact molecular copies, had adverse risks including higher risks of breast cancer, stroke, heart disease and blood clots than in non-users. Although the added risk was small many women stopped using HRT and more never took it up as a treatment option.

However, women continued to experience discomfort with menopause and this led to two different outcomes. One was the second wave of hormone use, termed hormone therapy (HT) and the other was a surge towards alternative remedies – that is, nutraceuticals.

The exogenous hormones prescribed in HT include oestrogen, progesterone and sometimes combined oestrogen and progesterone, and to address sexual issues, some testosterone treatments. The premise is that as the levels of all these hormones are lowering naturally in the body due to menopause, the prescribed hormones will top you up and remove menopause symptoms. How you get the external hormones into your system varies from pills, patches, gels, implants and pessaries. The other modification making doses more sensitive is whether the hormones are in a cyclical release, like the menstrual cycle, or continuous.

Which hormone therapy you select, and the best delivery method, will be determined by your individual needs, but with so many options it may take time to work through the relevant information. As well as consulting an expert in the field, I recommend learning as much as you can. If you have had hormone-driven cancer, or are at risk, HT will never be an option.

Starting HT once transition symptoms start and then gradually removing HT after a few years has been shown to be helpful for some women. A large review study examining the results of many clinical trials found that HT did reduce the frequency of hot flushes by up to seventy-five per cent compared to placebo; however, the placebo group also enjoyed a fifty-seven per cent reduction. The difference was only eighteen per cent, and while the placebo group had lower benefit they did escape the reported side effects of HT, which were breast tenderness, oedema, joint pain and psychological discomfort. Belief in symptom respite makes a profound difference to experience and confirms the important role of mindstyle.

Hormone therapy is also given to improve sexual function. An investigation into different forms of HT, such as oestrogens alone and oestrogens in combination with progestogens, considered the treatment benefits of over 16,000 women and found small to moderate reduction in pain related to sexual function when used at the onset of menopause or within the first five years only. The use of HT for sexual issues has the same adverse risks as its use to treat hot flushes. But there are site-specific oestrogen treatments to assist sexual function available that don't have the same adverse side effects. Vaginal oestriol is the weakest form of oestrogen and the one that specifically offers the most benefit for relief of vaginal dryness, as well as discomfort with sexual intercourse, wrinkles and maintaining bone density. This form of oestrogen does not impact the disease risks mentioned above as it is absorbed by the vaginal tissues.

There are also plenty of over-the-counter lubrication options but go for water-based vaginal lubricants and silicone-based lubricants or moisturisers. Try to avoid products that include glycerine, as it can cause burning or irritation in some women. Staying sexually active in any form also helps by increasing blood flow to the vagina.

Although HT does provide benefits, it also has adverse side effects like those reported above, and research over the past decade has tended to confirm the findings of the WHI and MWS that a standard dose of HT increases stroke risk to two strokes per 10,000, and that long-term use of hormones may increase cardiovascular, stroke and breast cancer risk. HT also increases mortality. We are all going to die at some stage but there is a small suggestion that HT may make it happen sooner. Only you know how much risk you want to tolerate and weigh that against the benefits for reducing menopause symptoms and improving your quality of life. Balance these facts up and sort out what will be right for you.

Bio-identical hormones

Due to the fallout from the medical research regarding HT, a more natural approach was developed in which hormones with identical molecular structures to our endogenous hormones were developed. In the past fifteen years the development and use of these products has grown exponentially and they are now termed body-identical hormone replacement treatment (BHRT). Although considered 'more natural', they are artificially made, with bio-identical oestrogen (17 beta oestradiol) being synthesised from a plant chemical extract; bio-identical progesterone is derived from micronised progesterone to make it more absorbable. This is noteworthy, as some of the criticism of HT in increasing breast cancer risk relates to synthetic progestogen.

What makes body-identical hormones 'natural' is that the body can't tell the difference between your endogenous hormones and these bio-identical exogenous ones, and they behave the same way in the body by attaching to oestrogen receptors and then turning them on just as your own oestrogen would. There is a range of bio-identical products including pills, patches, creams, capsules and gels.

It is recommended that for body-identical hormones to be safe and effective, and for them to be truly like the body, the hormone blood levels should be checked regularly so that the physiological quantities and properties and proportions of hormones can be monitored. Recall that our body is constantly monitoring hormone levels and adjusting accordingly, so the problem with adding in hormones, identical or otherwise, is that the natural balance system is overridden and there can be an increase in hormones which increases cancer risk. HT or use of bio-identical hormones is not a viable long-term solution because of the associated risks for breast cancer, stroke and thromboembolic disease. Review their use regularly and have a back-up plan if necessary.

Non-hormonal medications

Non-hormonal medications have been reportedly used to relieve menopausal symptoms, but there is a lack of quality medical reviews supporting their use. For example, anti-inflammatory agents have been used to counteract or suppress the inflammatory process – this includes non-steroidal anti-inflammatory drugs (NSAIDs). Like all medications they have a risk of side effects, even the newer generation ones. Adrenal blockers have also been used to reduce hot sweats, but they interfere with the adrenal system globally, which can be counterproductive as it serves multiple useful purposes, including the natural supply and conversion of androgen into oestrogen. This suggests that adrenal blockers may reduce your hot flushes but simultaneously reduce your available oestrogen.

One area where alternative medications are being used to treat symptoms for which they were not designed, and at levels causing increasing concern within psychiatry, is the use of psychotropic and serotonin-manipulating drugs for women in menopause. The argument for using these medications is that they can assist women for whom hormone therapy is not an option, such as women with breast cancer or high breast cancer risks. However, the argument against is that these medications have significant troublesome adverse side effects and have not been developed for the management of menopausal symptoms such as hot flushes. There is limited research specifically examining their benefits in treating symptoms, how they impact negatively, and how they compare to other interventions, including psychological therapies.

A large study that examined treatment trials of psychiatric medication's effects on hot flushes found that they were less effective than HT and that the adverse side effects and financial costs meant they were not particularly useful or practical for women who can take HT. But the conclusion was that they may offer some benefit for women who can't take HT and/or who have a mood disorder for which they were designed.

Psychotropic medications being (mis)used to treat menopausal symptoms include the family of antidepressants that influence the amount of circulating serotonin, known as Selective Serotonin Re-uptake Inhibitors (SSRIs), and the Serotonin Noradrenaline Re-uptake Inhibitors (SNRIs). They have been used to treat hot flushes despite their significant side effects, which may completely compromise quality of life and exacerbate other menopause symptoms such as loss of libido, weight gain and appetite changes. Another medication is Gabapentin, which is an anti-convulsant used to manage epilepsy. Reportedly it can improve hot flushes and night sweats, but side effects include sleeplessness. Imagine no night sweats but you can't sleep anyway and risk dizziness, weight gain, dry mouth and day-time sedation. Again, weigh up the pros and cons for your unique needs and discuss with at least one health professional, and actively monitor any drug's use and side effects.

In women with mood symptoms there is also concern that mood stabilisers and psychotropic medications may be over-prescribed to address phasic mood disturbance or psycho-social issues that are best suited to relationship counselling or other therapies and lifestyle changes, as previously described.

Psychological treatment

Non-pharmacological evidence-based treatments also include psycho-education and cognitive behaviour therapy (CBT). Providing women with information regarding the transition and symptoms has been found to be very effective at reducing discomfort and distress, partly by removing doubt and by validating of individual experience and the empowerment of self-knowledge. CBT, which is a psychological treatment model, is particularly efficacious at relieving mood symptoms and anxiety and reducing stress, which may indirectly help reduce hot flushes and sweats. CBT for depression and anxiety is found to be as effective as medication, and as there is nothing at all going into the body and changing its physiology, CBT does not have adverse health side effects. The benefits also tend to be much longer lasting after the end of treatment because CBT requires people to learn new strategies and ways to manage in life that transcend menopause.

Components of a psychological program for menopause may include education, relaxation techniques, sleep hygiene, developing a positive attitude, changing perceptions regarding symptoms, self-acceptance and goal setting.

Medical hypnotherapy may be applied within a psychological therapy or by a medical or other health practitioner and has many applications. It is sometimes offered to decrease the number of hot flushes, but we lack independent research indicating that it works. As with all complementary health service providers, please check that any treating medical practitioner or psychologist is qualified and registered.

Complementary and alternative health therapies

There are many other forms of therapy for managing menopause symptoms, and again hot flushes specifically. There are also many individuals and occupational groups presenting themselves as health therapists and experts in menopause. The list is growing exponentially now as more health practitioners recognise that menopause management has been a largely ignored consumer market.

Research suggests that few of the advertised services for managing menopause symptoms have the scientific evidence to back up their claims. Many of these services, just like health products, may have placebo effects or psychological benefits because you know you are doing something and that makes you feel better. That is okay, but the risk is that some may be expensive in terms of your time and money, and they may also distract you from more beneficial options or they may be potentially harmful.

There are several things you can do to help protect yourself from investing in an unhelpful service. First, check the qualifications of the service or therapy provider. Qualified health practitioners must be registered. In Australia, this is very easy to check, as there is one governing nationwide health practitioner regulatory body called the Australian Health Practitioner Regulation Agency (AHPRA. gov.au). This agency lists every registered health practitioner from optometrist to oncologist, podiatrist to psychologists, osteopath to Chinese medicine and acupuncture provider. There are other health providers who are registered with their own professional group, so check there too, but be mindful that because they are not with AHPRA they do not have a legally binding ethical code of conduct or statutory duty of care.

Second, getting another set of eyes on a problem is a good rule of thumb, and in health it usually means obtaining a second opinion. Be careful of practitioners pushing products. In some instances, they get commissions from the products they sell, so the more 'treatments' you purchase the more money they make. Think for a moment that doctors diagnose health issues but do not sell you medicine; you must buy your medicine from a pharmacist. This system was developed to prevent conflict of interest.

Third, be vigilant about the offered treatment. Do your research and investigate what the evidence says about the effectiveness of the treatment or service offered. Investigate how other people have responded to the service. However, as a health professional registered with AHPRA cannot use testimonials, you will need to ask how other people have responded to the treatment, what the common side effects or consequences are and how long the course of intervention or service usually lasts.

Acupuncture

The ancient practice of Chinese needle therapy is termed acupuncture. It is based on a theoretical understanding that disease processes influence the health of our body. It arose in the third century BC, so is over 10,000 years older than western medicine. According to the model every organ in the body has a meridian line of energy. There are yin and yang lines, and these are under the control of eight extraordinary meta-systems. The needle points, or acupuncture points, are at specific points in relation to other organs and meridians. Traditional treatment focuses on each specific symptom differentially, so there is no panacea or general treatment, rather a very individualised program of precise and specific symptom management. Western medicine is only now developing this individualised approach to treatment.

Acupuncture involves the insertion of very fine needles into specific points on the body and, unlike pharmacological and many other alternative or natural remedies, has very few adverse events or negative risks and side effects. Recently there has been considerable progress in western research understanding all the neural and physiological mechanisms involved in acupuncture to explain its effectiveness and its apparent analgesic effect. Specifically, acupuncture appears to modulate our naturally occurring opioids, serotonin and noradrenaline.

Menopause, like many other medical conditions, is experienced and expressed differently in Asian tradition than in western countries. Women have the same menopausal symptoms worldwide, but they are interpreted differently depending upon where you are from. According to Chinese medicine practice, menopause is a natural change in energy. The ovaries and uterus go together with the liver, spleen and kidneys in the pelvic region. Acupuncture has been found to successfully reduce multiple menopausal symptoms – for example, hot flushes and night sweats, insomnia and fatigue, mood swings, headaches, joint pain and heart palpitations. However, just like HT treatment, the topic is polarised. For example, two different menopause sites give contradictory messages, and some medical researchers and practitioners also have divergent views.

The peri-menopausal symptoms most commonly treated with acupuncture, and with research evidence to back it up, is hot flushes and nights sweats, which under western models are due to vasomotor changes (specifically the dilation of blood vessels in the skin). According to traditional Chinese medicine models, during menopause the yin depletion leads to a flare of yang which is a warming element but not a true heat. Thus, in Chinese medicine a hot flush is interpreted as an 'empty heat', as there is no inflammatory process. Hot flushes are not negatively perceived. The idea of acupuncture is to help rebalance the flow of energy – to assist the change of heat from the pelvis to the heart.

Recent research suggests that we have a thermal-neutral zone (TNZ), which is the tolerable temperature zone between the environment and core body temperature. When this neutral zone is breached, we may sweat and flush, and unfortunately during menopause, for women experiencing vasomotor symptoms this zone narrows, making them more susceptible to hot flushes and sweats. Acupuncture within westernised models is believed to work by re-normalising the TNZ.

A twelve-week study from Norway found that women who received acupuncture experienced a decline in both number and intensity of hot flushes per day. In another study, twenty-seven women were given true acupuncture involving the placement of needles at specific sites to boost energy and release endorphins for ten weeks. Their scores on symptoms rating scales were then compared with those of twenty-six women who received fake acupuncture (blunt needles below stimulation threshold). The women with the real treatment had less frequent and less intense hot flushes and additionally reported fewer mood symptoms. Importantly, a 2016 study of more than two hundred women experiencing a minimum of four hot flushes per night, with either six or twelve months of treatment, found that maximum benefit occurred after about eight treatments. It is worth noting that frequency of night sweats decreased by thirty per cent, meaning that on average women experienced one and a bit fewer events each night.

Acupuncture has also been found to be effective for the treatment of the psychological discomfort of anxiety and depression – not just in menopausal women, but in all adults diagnosed with those mental illnesses.

There are different acupuncture processes and a diverse number of target points, but one thing is consistent, and that is the need for regular long-term intervention, as with other forms of treatment. Acupuncture is not a one jab option. The guidelines suggest that you have an intense course at the start and then monthly treatments to maintain benefits. For example, an early study found that initial sessions were necessary two to three times per week, then monthly for a year, with sessions every two months thereafter until post-menopause was helpful for the reduction of hot flushes.

A significant investigation of multiple acupuncture trials was unable to find any evidence for, or against, the benefits of acupuncture in controlling vasomotor symptoms compared to sham or placebo treatment. It was, however, better than doing nothing and, although less effective than HT, acupuncture does not have the adverse consequences for longer term health risks.

Case study: Open minded

I think I was forty-eight or forty-nine when I entered peri-menopause. What I noticed first was the irregularity of my periods: they were more spaced apart and a lot heavier. I thought, What's all this about? as I had definitely had no issues ever before with them.

They were heavier for about a year to a point that I was getting frustrated, as they could happen any place anywhere, and this was hard to manage in my head and practically – especially as I work.

Then in early summer I noticed mild surges in heat during the day, and a few times at night I would wake up with the extra heat. I had never been a hot person, in fact I always suffer from the cold, and thought, Terrific that's going to be great, but it became an annoyance.

We then went to Japan for holidays and again I thought, Great I will keep warmer, and it was true that the heat surges were not quite as obvious in the cold. But returning to the Aussie summer I would experience flushes two or three times a night and I would wake, and then generally being hot and the heat of the weather would stop me from falling back to sleep.

My sleep was disturbed, so I felt I was walking around quite sleep deprived. I had no period for three months and then five months and thought, Great this is over, but no it reappeared again. I was hoping it was all over. After the five-month break between periods, I had a regular period, then twenty-two days later had a super-heavy period. Very annoying!

I also noticed that the hot flushes were preceded by a nauseated feeling in my stomach for five to ten seconds. This is not ideal in my line of work as I work one on one with people and going red in the face, feeling sick and getting hot is not good when clients are right in front of you. I managed by opening the office window and wearing layers of clothing I could take off – so I take layers off and put them back on and I don't think people really notice.

I basically ignored my symptoms as I didn't want necessarily to take HRT. At night the nausea was waking me before the hot flush and the sleep deprivation was becoming a big problem. I also felt my memory was not so good, I was forgetting things, not on the ball, trouble finding words, and my mood was getting crotchety and I am always a happy up-beat person.

I spoke to my GP and had told her I don't want hormones. I am not a person to pop a pill to sort problems.

She suggested I try acupuncture. I had always thought acupuncture was for sore muscles, but I went to the first session with an open mind and lots of questions. The acupuncturist explained they could turn up or down the heat in organs, which was all news to me. I had twelve needles. For the next day and a half, I did not have a hot flush at all, then they returned but not as frequently and not as intense. Following the second session they pretty much disappeared. It was subtle. I had no nausea in my stomach and the fatigue gradually left.

It probably took a month to feel better. All nausea is gone, all heat is gone, but I still wake around three am.

*What I am left with long term is having to manage sleep.
I go to bed early around nine-thirty because I sleep best in
the first section, so I get a solid sleep before I wake. For the
time being I am seeing the acupuncturist weekly, however
his plan is to reduce that as my body adjusts – not sure how
long that will take.*

*I would say things are manageable, but I would be panic
stricken if I could not get to the acupuncturist every week.
I also have this uneasiness as I don't know what is ahead of
me – will it reach a crescendo and get worse or am I over
the worst already? It does sit on my mind that I don't know
when it will end or if it will get worse. I will just get help as
I go if necessary.*

Summary: Choosing your best management strategies

- **Be an individual.** We are all unique, so it is important
  that we honour our uniqueness, have an individualised
  approach to our health care and have the capacity and
  options to make the best choices for ourselves. Explore
  all your options with your health practitioner/s and get a
  program tailored just for you.
- **Be informed and informative.** Understand that every
  treatment option has consequences and appreciate that
  doing nothing has consequences too. Be aware of all the
  adverse effects and risks of treatments prescribed, 'natural'
  and so forth. Inform all treating health practitioners what
  you are taking and doing in terms of lifestyle to optimise
  all benefits and reduce potential harm.
- **Go natural first.** Menopause is a natural process and
  it is possible it will pass without the hype, drama and
  discomfort you may hear so much about. Allow your
  menopause transition to unfold naturally and then add

269

in treatment as necessary. Start by exploring lifestyle changes first and then add more interventions if needed.

- **Manage and monitor.** Actively manage your symptoms if they cause discomfort or distress, so that things do not spiral badly and severely impact upon your quality of life. Because the transition changes, monitor and review your treatment strategies to see if they are still helpful or need augmenting.

- **Pause and trust yourself.** Take the time to engage with your inner self, to read and understand your body's signs and signals. Then support yourself to make the best decision and take the optimal path forwards. Your body trusts your brain to take care of it.

Final Words

Menopause is a natural stage in our lives, as our entire being adjusts to a lowering of hormones necessary for sexual reproductive function into levels required for health maintenance. Menopause marks a major transition and heralds a new transformative autonomy for women.

Embrace yourself. Listen to your body and inner wisdom. Hear its signals but don't rush – relax and allow menopause to unfold by supporting your physical and mental wellbeing. Consider all options before you medicate or replace hormones without first identifying or addressing the underlying cause of your distress. It might not be due to hormonal loss: it could be the need to improve your relationship, learn how to care for yourself, develop a healthy lifestyle or develop a positive mindstyle.

Be kind to yourself if you find you need assistance, and learn what helps you to be comfortable – it is never a failure to need help. A significant number of women do want some form of physical relief from menopausal discomfort, whether it be through lifestyle changes, supplements, acupuncture or medication, and that need is natural. You also don't need to wait until you feel overwhelmed or until you are in menopause. If necessary, start intervention in peri-menopause, as there is evidence to suggest that the change in hormone ratio is more of an issue than the final cessation. Just start gently, take any medications or supplements in low doses and slowly increase the dose to take the edge off, and plan to review the intervention within five years.

Understand that the biochemical and hormonal make-up of your body is influenced by your thoughts and emotional wellbeing as well as your health. Check your perceptions and attitudes towards yourself, menopause, age and life, as what goes on in your mind impacts every cell in your body. Your beliefs are possibly more powerful than your genes because your thoughts either increase the sympathetic nervous system stress response or soothe it. Engaging the parasympathetic system is vital for restoration. Find your inner language so your mind speaks kindly and helpfully to your body.

Become self-compassionate and learn to love yourself and those parts of you that you feel critical of or find unacceptable or a failure or an imperfection. Practise the art of self-acceptance. Also, to go forwards without burden, it is necessary to have forgiveness and let go of the past. Stop avoiding those feelings and memories that are unpleasant. Carrying negative painful emotions or unfinished emotional processing affects your body, so rather than continuing to avoid emotional pains, face them – that is the way they pass. Welcome them into your life story and consider what you learned, as those experiences are aspects that shaped you and helped you grow into the amazing wonderful woman you are today. Accept yourself unconditionally.

Build your midlife foundation, as this is where you will grow from and this will contribute to your late-life wellbeing. Love who you are and identify what you want so you can set new intentions and make the best choices. Consider all aspects of your life – physical and mental health, relationships, occupation or vocation, financial security, environment, leisure, spirituality and meaning, and purpose. Find your passion/s and what makes your soul sing, as having goals will re-energise you. Make a commitment to always cherish and honour yourself to help you flourish for the next third of your life.

References

PART 1

Austad, SN. (1994). 'Menopause: an evolutionary perspective'. *Experimental Gerontology* 29(3–4): 255–63

Beery, AK., & Zucker, I. (2011). 'Sex bias in neuroscience and biomedical research'. *Neuroscience and Behavioral Reviews* 35: 565–72

Brizendine, L. (2006). *The female brain*. Broadway Books. United States of America

Clayton, JA., & Collins, FS. (2014). 'Policy: NIH to balance sex in cell and animal studies'. *Nature* 509(7500): 282–3

Epperson, CN., et al. (2013). 'Menopause effects on verbal memory: findings from a longitudinal community cohort'. *The Journal of Clinical Endocrinology and Metabolism* 98(9): 3829–38

Gooren, LJ., & Giltay, EJ. (2014). 'Men and women, so different, so similar: observations from cross-sex hormone treatment of transsexual subjects'. *Andrologia* 46(5): 570–5

Holdcroft, A. (2007). 'Gender bias in research: how does it affect evidence-based medicine?'. *The Journal of the Royal Society of Medicine* Jan; 100(1): 2–3

Kandel, E., et al. (1991). *Principles of neuroscience* 3rd edition. Prentice Hall International

Keville, TD. (1994). 'The invisible woman: gender bias in medical research'. *Women's Rights. Law Reporter* 15: 123–42

Koebele, S.V., et al. (2017). 'Cognitive changes across the menopause transition: a longitudinal evaluation of the impact of age and ovarian status on spatial memory'. *Hormones and Behavior* 87: 96–114

McCarthy, M. (2015). 'Sex differences in the brain'. *The Scientist* Oct; 1: 306–21

Micale, MS. (1993). 'On the "disappearance" of hysteria: a study in the clinical deconstruction of a diagnosis'. *Isis* 84(3): 496–526

Polachek, I., et al. (2017). 'Sex differences in psychiatric hospitalizations of individuals with psychotic disorders'. *The Journal of Nervous and Mental Disease* 205(4): 313–17

Ruigrok, ANV. (2014). 'A meta-analysis of sex differences in human brain structure'. *Neuroscience and Behavioral Reviews* 39(100): 34–50

Shi L., et al. (2016). 'Sex biased gene expression profiling of human brains at major developmental stages'. *Scientific Reports* 6: article number 21181

Skolund, C., et al. (2016). 'Association of hormonal contraception with depression'. *JAMA Psychiatry* 73(11): 1154–62

Stevenson, B., & Wolfers, J. (2009). 'The paradox of declining female happiness'. *American Economic Journal: Economic Policy* 1(2): 190–225

Tasca, C., et al. (2012). 'Women and hysteria in the history of mental health'. *Clinical Practice & Epidemiology in Mental Health* 8: 110–19

Upadhayay, N., & Guragain, S. (2014). 'Comparison of cognitive functions between male and female medical students: a pilot study'. *Journal of Clinical and Diagnostic Research* 8(6): BC12–BC15

Van Goozen, SH., et al. (1950). 'Gender differences in behaviour: activating effects of cross-sex hormones'. *Psychoneuroendocrinology* 20(4): 343–63

Van Goozen, SH., et al. (2002). 'Organizing and activating effects of sex hormones in homosexual transsexuals'. *Behavioral Neuroscience* 116(6): 982–8

Part 2

Cassar, S., et al. (2016). 'Insulin resistance in polycystic ovary syndrome: a systematic review and meta-analysis of euglycaemic–hyperinsulinaemic clamp studies'. *Human Reproduction* 31(11): 2619–31

Chen, G., et al. (2014). 'Associations between sleep duration, daytime nap duration, and osteoporosis vary by sex, menopause, and sleep quality'. *The Journal of Clinical Endocrinology and Metabolism* 99:8 2869–77

Falcone, T., et al (1992). 'Impaired glucose effectiveness in patients with polycystic ovary syndrome'. *Human Reproduction* 7(7): 922–5

Faubion, SS. (2016). *The menopause solution.* Mayo Foundation for Medical Education and Research. Time Inc Books

Freedman, RR. (2014). 'Menopause and sleep'. *Menopause* 21(5): 534–5

Freedman, RR., & Roehrs, TA. (2007). 'Sleep disturbance in menopause'. *Menopause* 14(5) 826–9

Gill, J. (2000). 'The effects of moderate alcohol consumption on female hormone levels and reproductive function'. *Alcohol and Alcoholism* 35(5): 417–23

Gupte, AA., et al. (2015). 'Estrogen: an emerging regulator of insulin action and mitochondrial function'. *Journal of Diabetes Research* article ID 916585

Krassas, GE., & Papadopoulou, P. (2001). 'Review article: oestrogen action on bone cells'. *Journal of Musculoskeletal and Neuronal Interactions* 2(2): 143–51

Nestler, JE. (1997). 'Insulin regulation of human ovarian androgens'. *Human Reproduction* 12 (suppl 1): 53–62

Scheen, AJ. (1997). 'Perspective in the treatment of insulin resistance'. *Human Reproduction* 12 (suppl 1): 63–71

Schliep, KC., et al. (2015). Alcohol intake, reproductive hormones, and menstrual cycle function: a prospective cohort study'. *The American Journal of Clinical Nutrition* 102(4): 933–42

The Amsterdam ESHRE/ASRM-Sponsored 3rd PCOS Consensus Workshop Group. (2012). 'Consensus on women's health aspects of polycystic ovary syndrome (PCOS)'. *Human Reproduction* 27(1): 14–24

Part 3

Azam, M.N., et al. (1995). 'Spontaneous coronary artery dissection associated with oral contraceptive use'. *The International Journal of Cardiology* Feb; 48(2): 195–8

Bittner, V. (2009). 'Menopause, age, and cardiovascular risk: a complex relationship'. *Journal of the American College of Cardiology* 54: 2374–5

Chen, G., et al. (2014). 'Associations between sleep duration, daytime nap duration, and osteoporosis vary by sex, menopause, and sleep quality'. *The Journal of Clinical Endocrinology and Metabolism* 99(8) 2869–77

Collaborative Group on Hormonal Factors in Breast Cancer (2012). 'Menarche, menopause, and breast cancer risk: individual participant meta-analysis, including 118,964 women with breast cancer from 117 epidemiological studies'. *The Lancet Oncology* 13(11): 1141–51

de Kat, AC., et al (2017). 'Unravelling the associations of age and menopause with cardiovascular risk factors in a large population-based study'. *BMC Medicine* 15: 2

Doshi, SB., & Agarwa, A. (2013). 'The role of oxidative stress in menopause'. *Journal of Mid-Life Health* 4(3): 140–6

Erlanger, D., et al. (1999). 'Hormones and cognition: current concepts and issues in neuropsychology'. *Neuropsychology Review* 9(4): 175–207

Faubion, SS. (2016). *The menopause solution*. Mayo Foundation for Medical Education and Research. Time Inc Books

Faubion, SS., et al. (2015). 'Long-term health consequences of premature or early menopause and considerations for management'. *Climacteric* 18(4): 483–91

Freeman, DE., & Sherfi, K. (2007). 'Prevalence of hot flushes and night sweats around the world: a systematic review'. *Climacteric* 3: 197–214

Freedman, RR. (2014). 'Menopause and sleep'. *Menopause* 21(5): 534–5

Freedman, RR., & Roehrs, TA. (2004). 'Lack of sleep disturbance from menopausal hot flushes'. *Fertility and Sterility* 82(1): 138–44

Freedman, RR., & Roehrs, TA. (2007). 'Sleep disturbance in menopause'. *Menopause* 14(5): 826–9

Gupte, AA., et al. (2015). 'Estrogen: an emerging regulator of insulin action and mitochondrial function'. *Journal of Diabetes Research* Article ID 916585

Khan K., et al. (2018). 'Difference in management and outcomes for men and women with ST-elevations myocardial infarction'. *Medical Journal of Australia* published online 23 Jul; doi: 10.5694/mja17.01109

Krassas, GE., & Papadopoulou, P. (2001). 'Review article. oestrogen action on bone cells'. *Journal of Musculoskeletal and Neuronal Interactions* 2(2): 143–51

Kravitz, HM, et al. (2008). 'Sleep disturbance during the menopausal transition in a multi-ethnic community sample of women'. *Sleep* 31(7): 979–90

Lindor, RA., et al. (2016). 'Emergency department presentation of patients with spontaneous coronary artery dissection'. *Journal of Emergency Medicine* S0736–4679(16): 30716–8

McGrath-Cadell, L., et al. (2016). 'Outcomes of patients with spontaneous coronary artery dissection'. *Open Heart* 3(2): e000491

Mayor, S. (2016). 'Early menopause is linked to higher risk of cardiovascular disease and death'. *BMJ* (Clinical research ed.) 354: i5004

National Cancer Institute. 'Alcohol and cancer risk'. <cancer.gov/about-cancer/causes-prevention/risk/alcohol/alcohol-fact-sheet>

Nelson, LM. (2009). 'Primary ovarian insufficiency'. *The New England Journal of Medicine* 360(6): 606–14

Park, C., et al. (2009). 'Premature menopause linked to CVD and osteoporosis'. *The Journal of Clinical Endocrinology and Metabolism* 94: 4953–60

Rindner, L. (2017). 'Reducing menopausal symptoms for women during the menopause transition using group education in a primary health care setting – a randomized controlled trial'. *Maturitas* 88: 14–19

Ripa, P., et al. (2015). 'Migraine in menopausal women: a systematic review'. *The International Journal of Women's Health* 7: 773–82

Svejme, O., et al. (2012). 'Early menopause and risk of osteoporosis, fracture and mortality: a 34-year prospective observational study in 390 women'. *BJOG* 119: 810–16

Tao, XY., et al. (2016). 'Effect of primary ovarian insufficiency and early natural menopause on mortality: a meta-analysis'. *Climacteric* 19(1): 27–36

Part 4

Avis, N. (1994). 'A longitudinal analysis of the association between menopause and depression. Results from the Massachusetts women's health study'. *Annals of Epidemiology* 4(3): 214–20

Ayers, B., et al. (2010). 'The impact of attitudes towards the menopause on women's symptom experience: systematic review'. *Maturitas* Jan; 65(1): 28–36

Ayers, B., et al. (2013). 'Health related quality of life of women with menopausal hot flushes and night sweats'. *Climacteric* Apr; 16(2): 235–9

Bale, TL., & Epperson, CN. (2015). 'Sex differences and stress across the lifespan'. *Nature Neuroscience* 18(10): 1413–20

Banis, S., et al. (2014). 'Acute stress modulates feedback processing in men and women: differential effects on the feedback-related negativity and Theta and Beta power'. *PLoS ONE* 9(4): e95690

Barth, C., et al. (2016). 'In-vivo dynamics of the human hippocampus across the menstrual cycle'. *Scientific Reports* 7(6): 32833

Brinton, RD. (2016). 'Neuro-endocrinology: oestrogen therapy affects brain structure but not function'. *Nature Reviews Neurology* 12(10): 561–2

Brinton, RD., et al. (2008). 'Progesterone receptors: form and function in brain'. *Frontiers in Neuroendocrinology* 29: 313–39

Cavill, R., et al (2014). 'The effects of menstrual-related pain on attentional interference'. *Pain* 155(4): 821–7

Chauchan, A., et al. (2017). 'Sex differences in ischaemic stroke: potential cellular mechanisms'. *Clinical Science* 31(7): 533–52

Chibber, A., et al. (2017). 'Estrogen receptor β deficiency impairs BDNF-5-HT signaling in the hippocampus of female brain: a possible mechanism for menopausal depression'. *Psychoneuroendocrinology* 82: 107–16

Clayton, JA., & Collins, FS. (2014). 'Policy: NIH to balance sex in cell and animal studies'. *Nature.* 509(7500): 282–3

Doshi, SB., & Agarwal, A. (2013). 'The role of oxidative stress in menopause'. *Journal of Mid-life Health* 4: 140–6

Epperson, CN., et al. (2013). 'Menopause effects on verbal memory: findings from a longitudinal community cohort'. *The Journal of Clinical Endocrinology and Metabolism* 98: 3829–38

Fink, G., et al. (1996). 'Estrogen control of central neurotransmission: effect on mood, mental state, and memory'. *Cellular and Molecular Neurobiology* Jun; 16(3): 325–44

Galvan, T., et al. (2017). 'Association of estradiol with sleep apnoea in depressed perimenopausal and postmenopausal women: a preliminary study'. *Menopause* 24(1): 112–17

Gillies, GE., & McArthur, S. (2010). 'Estrogen actions in the brain and the basis for differential action in men and women: a case for sex-specific medicines'. *Pharmacological Reviews* Jun; 62(2): 155–98

Gordon, JL., et al. (2016). 'Naturally occurring changes in estradiol concentrations in the menopause transition predict morning cortisol and negative mood in perimenopausal depression'. *Clinical Psychological Science* 4(5): 919–35

Hagemann, G., et al. (2011). 'Changes in brain size during the menstrual cycle'. *PLoS One* 6(2): e14655

Hall, E., & Steiner, M. (2013). 'Serotonin and female psychopathology'. *Women's Health London* Jan; 9(1): 85–97

Hay, M. (2015). 'Sex, the brain and hypertension: brain oestrogen receptors and high blood pressure risk factors'. *Clinical Science* 130(1): 9–18

Holland, J. (2015). 'Medicating women's feelings'. *New York Times* 28 Feb

Honman, H., et al. (2017). 'Estrogen-related factors in the frontal lobe of Alzheimer's disease patients and importance of body mass index'. *Science Reports* 7(1): 726

Imtiaz, B. (2017). 'Postmenopausal hormone therapy and Alzheimer disease: a prospective cohort study'. *Neurology* 14 Mar; 88(11): 1062–8

Imtiaz, B., et al (2017). 'Risk of Alzheimer's disease among users of postmenopausal hormone therapy: a nationwide case-control study'. *Maturitas* Apr; 98: 7–13

Janicki, SC., & Schupf, N. (2010). 'Hormonal influences on cognition and risk for Alzheimer disease'. *Current Neurology and Neuroscience Reports* Sep; 10(5): 359–66

Jernigan, TL., et al. (2011). 'Postnatal brain development: structural imaging of dynamic neurodevelopmental processes'. *Progress in Brain Research* 189: 77–92

Karim, R., et al. (2016). 'Effect of reproductive history and exogenous hormone use on cognitive function in mid- and late life'. *Journal of the American Geriatrics Society* 64(12): 2448–56

Kenealy, BP., et al. (2013). 'Neuroestradiol in the hypothalamus contributes to the regulation of gonadotropin releasing hormone release'. *Journal of Neuroscience* 33(49): 190051–9

Kocoska-Maras, L., et al. (2013). 'Cognitive function in association with sex hormones in postmenopausal women'. *Gynecological Endocrinology* 29(1): 59–62

Koebele, S., et al. (2017). 'Cognitive changes across the menopause transition: a longitudinal evaluation of the impact of age and ovarian status on spatial memory'. *Hormones and Behavior* 87: 96–114

Leuner, B., et al (2014). 'Chronic gestational stress leads to depressive-like behavior and compromises medial prefrontal cortex structure and function during the postpartum period'. *PLoS One* 9(3): e89912

Li, R., et al. (2014). 'Brain sex matters: estrogen in cognition and Alzheimer's disease'. *Molecular and Cellular Endocrinology* 25 May; 389(1–2): 13–21

Lokuge, S., et al. (2010). 'The rapid effects of estrogen: a mini-review'. *Behavioural Pharmacology* 21: 465–72

Marjoribanks, J., et al. (2012). 'Long-term hormone therapy for peri-menopausal and menopausal women'. *Cochrane Database of Systematic Reviews* 11(7): CD004143

Mishra, GD., et al. (2003). 'Physical and mental health: changes during the menopause transition'. *Quality of Life Research* 12: 405

Novais, A., et al. (2017). 'How age, sex and genotype shape the stress response'. *Neurobiology of Stress* Feb; 6: 44–56

Olofsson, AS., & Collins, A. (2000). 'Psychosocial factors, attitude to menopause and symptoms in Swedish perimenopausal women'. *Climacteric* Mar; 3(1): 33–42

Oomen, CA., et al. (2009). 'Opposite effects of early maternal deprivation on neurogenesis in male versus female rats'. *PLoS One* 4(1): e3675

Osmanovic-Barilar, J., & Salkovic-Petrisi, M. (2016). 'Evaluating the role of hormone therapy in postmenopausal women with Alzheimer's disease'. *Drugs & Aging* 33(1): 787–808

Osterlund, MK., & Hurd, YL. (2001). 'Estrogen receptors in the human forebrain and the relation to neuropsychiatric disorders'. *Progress in Neurobiology* Jun; 64(3): 251–67

Petrovska, S., et al. (2012). 'Estrogens: mechanisms of neuroprotective effects'. *The Journal of Physiology and Biochemistry* Sep; 68(3): 455–60

Pines, A. (2016). 'Alzheimer's disease, menopause, and the impact of the estrogenic environment'. *Climacteric* 19(5): 430–2

Prokai, D., & Berga, SL. (2016). 'Neuroprotection via reduction in stress: altered menstrual patterns as a marker for stress and implications for long-term neurologic health in women'. *The International Journal of Molecular Sciences* 17(12): 2147

Rabot, S., et al. (2016). 'Impact of the gut microbiota on the neuroendocrine and behavioural responses to stress in rodents'. *OCL* 23(1): D116

Rettberg, JR., et al. (2014). 'Estrogen: a master regulator of bioenergetic systems in the brain and body'. *Frontiers in Neuroendocrinology* 35(1): 8–30

Rihender, L., et al. (2017). 'Reducing menopausal symptoms for women during the menopause transition using group education in a primary health care setting – a randomized controlled trial'. *Maturitas* Apr; 98: 14–19

Ryaczyk, LA., et al. (2005). 'An overlooked connection: serotonergic mediation of oestrogen-related physiology and pathology'. *BMC Women's Health* 5: 12

Soares, CN. (2011). 'In the heat of the moment: assessing anxiety and hot flushes in postmenopausal women'. *Menopause* 18(2): 121–2

Soares, CN. (2017). 'Tailoring strategies for the management of depression in midlife years'. *Menopause* 24(6): 699–701

Soni, M., et al. (2014). 'Phytoestrogens and cognitive function: a review'. *Maturitas* 77(3): 209–20

Syan, SK., et al. (2017). 'Influence of endogenous estradiol, progesterone, allopregnanolone, and dehydroepiandrosterone sulfate on brain resting state functional connectivity across the menstrual cycle'. *Fertility and Sterility* May; 107(5): 1246–55

Toffoletto, S., et al. (2008). 'Emotional and cognitive functional imaging of estrogen and progesterone effects in the female human brain: a systematic review'. *Psychoneuroendocrinology* 50: 28–52

Weiser, MJ., et al. (2008). 'Estrogen receptor beta in the brain: from form to function'. *Brain Research Reviews* 57: 309–20

Whittaker, J., et al. (2016). 'Gendered responses to the 2009 Black Saturday bushfires in Victoria, Australia. *Geographical Research* 54(2): 203–15

Yankova, M., et al. (2000). 'Estrogen increases synaptic connectivity between single pre-synaptic inputs and multiple post synaptic CA1 pyramidal cells: a serial electron-microscopic study'. *PNAS* 13 Mar; 98(6): 3525–30

Part 5

Aimé, C., et al. (2017). 'Grand mothering and cognitive resources are required for the emergence of menopause and extensive post-reproductive lifespan'. *PLoS Computational Biology* 20 Jul; 13(7): e1005631

Australian Social Trends 2014, reference 4102.0

Calleja-Agius, J., & Brincat, MP. (2015). 'The urogenital system and the menopause'. *Climacteric* 18(Suppl 1): 18–22

Champagne, FA., & Curley, JP. (2016). 'Plasticity of the maternal brain across the lifespan'. *New Directions for Child and Adolescent Development* 153: 9–21

Fenton, A., & Panay, N. (2014). 'Menopause and the workplace'. *Climacteric* 17(4): 317–18

Fisher, HE. (1998). 'Defining the brain systems of lust, romantic attraction and attachment'. *Human Nature* 9(1): 23–52

Gavin, R., et al. (2016). 'Menopause in the workplace: what employers should be doing'. *Maturitas* 85: 88–95

Mishra, GD., et al. (2003). 'Physical and mental health: changes during menopause transition'. *Quality of Life Research* 12: 405

Northrup, C. (2012). *The wisdom of menopause*. Bantam Books. New York

Payne S., & Doyal, L. (2010). 'Older women, work and health'. *Occupational Medicine* 60(3): 172–7

Rindner, L. (2017). 'Reducing menopausal symptoms for women during the menopause transition using group education in a primary health care setting – a randomized controlled trial'. *Maturitas* 98: 14–19

Roepe, L. (2015). 'Are Gen X women being squeezed out of the workplace?'. *Future of Work*. <www.fastcompany.com/3054410/ are-gen-x-women-being-squeezed-out-of-the-workplace>

Sarrel, P., et al (2015). 'Incremental direct and indirect costs of untreated vasomotor symptoms'. *Menopause* 22(3): 260–6

Sharron et al. (2000). 'Intimacy, commitment, and adaptation: sexual relationships within long-term marriages'. *Journal of Social and Personal Relationships* 21(5): 595–609

Solin, K. (2016). 'A bridge over troubled water'. *Huffington Post* 11 Nov

Vaughn, K., et al. (2017). 'Marriage, stress and menopause: midlife challenges and joys'. *The Journal of Sexual Medicine* 14(5): 675–86

Worsley, R., et al. (2012). 'Prevalence and predictors of low sexual desire, sexually related personal distress, and hypoactive sexual desire dysfunction in a community-based sample of midlife women'. *The Journal of Sexual Medicine* 10(1): 36–49

Part 6

Al-Saqi, SH., et al. (2015). 'Intravaginally applied oxytocin improves post-menopausal vaginal atrophy'. *Post Reproductive Health* 21(3): 88–97

Archer, DF., et al. (2011). 'Menopausal hot flushes and night sweats: where are we now?'. *Climacteric* 14: 515–28

Archer, DF., & Oger, E. (2012). 'Estrogen and progestogen effect on venous thromboembolism in menopausal women'. *Climacteric* 15: 235–40

Avis, NE., et al. (2016). 'Acupuncture in menopause (AIM) study: a pragmatic, randomized controlled trial'. *Menopause* 23(6): 626–37

Beral, V., & Million Women Study Collaborators. (2003). 'Breast cancer and hormone-replacement therapy in the Million Women Study'. *Lancet* 362(9382): 419–27

Borrelli, F, & Ernst, E. (2010). 'Alternative and complementary therapies for the menopause'. *Maturitas* 66: 333–43

Burrell, BA. (2009). 'The replacement of the replacement in menopause: hormone therapy, controversies, truth and risk'. *Nursing Inquiry* 16(3): 212–22

Chen, MN., et al. (2015). 'Efficacy of phytoestrogens for menopausal symptoms: a meta-analysis and systematic review'. *Climacteric* 18(2): 260–9

Chiu, HY., et al. (2015). 'Effects of acupuncture on menopause-related symptoms and quality of life in women in natural menopause: a meta-analysis of randomized controlled trials'. *Menopause* 22(2): 234–44

Cho, SH., & Whang, WW. (2009). 'Acupuncture for vasomotor menopausal symptoms: a systematic review'. *Menopause* 16(5): 1065–73

Dodin, S., et al. (2013). 'Acupuncture for menopausal hot flushes'. *Cochrane Database of Systematic Reviews* 30(7): CD007410

Gompel, A., & Santen, RJ. (2012). 'Hormone therapy and breast cancer risk 10 years after the WHI'. *Climacteric* 15: 241–9

Hall, E., et al. (2011). 'Non-hormonal treatment strategies for vasomotor symptoms: a critical review'. *Drugs* 71: 287–304

Henderson, VW., & Lobo, RA. (2012). 'Hormone therapy and the risk of stroke: perspectives 10 years after the Women's Health Initiative trials'. *Climacteric* 15: 229–34

Leach, MJ., & Moore, V. (2012). 'Black cohosh (Cimicifuga spp.) for menopausal symptoms'. *Cochrane Database of Systematic Reviews* 9: CD007244

Lethaby, A., et al. (2013). 'Phytoestrogens for menopausal vasomotor symptoms'. *Cochrane Database of Systematic Reviews* 10(12): CD001395

MacLennan, A., et al. (2004). 'Oral oestrogen and combined oestrogen/progestogen therapy versus placebo for hot flushes'. *Cochrane Database of Systematic Reviews* 18(4): CD002978

Mahmud, K. (2010). 'Natural hormone therapy for menopause'. *Gynecological Endocrinology* 26(2): 81–5

Mahmud, K. (2011). 'Hormones and breast cancer: can we use them in ways that could reduce the risk?'. *Oncology Reviews* 2(3): 146–53

Maki, PM. (2012). 'Hormone therapy, dementia, and cognition: the Women's Health Initiative 10 years on'. *Climacteric* 15: 256–62

Nastri, C., et al. (2013). 'Hormone therapy for sexual function in perimenopausal and postmenopausal women'. *Cochrane Database of Systematic Reviews* 6: CD009672

Pirotta, M. (2014). 'Acupuncture for menopausal vasomotor symptoms: study protocol for a randomised controlled trial'. *Trials* 15: 2241

Rada, G., et al. (2016). 'Non-hormonal interventions for hot flushes in women with a history of breast cancer'. *Cochrane Database of Systematic Reviews* 9: CD004923

Ronis, MJJ., et al (2018). 'Adverse effects of nutraceuticals and dietary supplements'. *Annual Review of Pharmacology and Toxicology* 58: 583–601

Rosenberg, K. (2016). 'Acupuncture relieves menopause-related vasomotor symptoms'. *American Journal of Nursing* 116(9): 68

Sharon, D., et al. (2007). 'The effect of dietary intake on hot flushes in menopausal women'. *The Journal of Obstetric, Gynecologic, & Neonatal Nursing* 36(3): 255–62

Stuenkel, CA., et al. (2015). 'Treatment of symptoms of the menopause: an endocrine society clinical practice guideline'. *The Journal of Clinical Endocrinology and Metabolism* 100(11): 3975–4011

Taku, K., et al. (2012). 'Extracted or synthesized soybean isoflavones reduce menopausal hot flash'. *Menopause* 19: 776–90

Trimarco, V., et al (2016). 'Effects of a new combination of nutraceuticals on postmenopausal symptoms and metabolic profile: a crossover, randomized, double-blind trial'. *International Journal of Women's Health* 8: 581–587

Van der Sluijs, CP., et al. (2007). 'Women's health during mid-life survey: the use of complementary and alternative medicine by symptomatic women transitioning through menopause in Sydney'. *Menopause* 14: 397–403

Wright, JV. (2005). 'Bio-identical steroid hormone replacement: selected observations from 23 years of clinical and laboratory practice'. *Annals of the New York Academy of Sciences* 1057(1): 506–24

Writing Group for the Women's Health Initiative Investigators (2002). 'Risks and benefit of estrogen plus progestin in healthy postmenopausal women: principal results from the Women's Health Initiative Randomized Controlled Trial'. *JAMA* 288: 321–333

Zhu, X., et al. (2016). 'Chinese herbal medicine for menopausal symptoms'. *Cochrane Database of Systematic Reviews* 15;3: CD009023

Acknowledgements

I wrote this book for my female friends and clients. Thank you for your faith in me and your excitement and enthusiasm to know more about yourselves. I hope this helps you to unravel the knots of the menopause transition and restore your hope and vitality for your future.

All the women who have ever entrusted me with your secrets and included me in part of your life journeys, thank you. I am honoured that you shared your experiences with me.

To the storytellers included in this book, I deeply appreciate the gift of your words and thank you for your honesty and generous support. May you know yourselves a little better, become kinder to yourselves and transform your lives.

For all the wonderful women I have had the pleasure to meet and for those who will discover this book, this is our story. Our bodies and brains are wonderful, complex and amazing. Let's be friends with ourselves, love generously, and thrive.

Lastly, thank you to my literary agent, editors and publisher for embracing this topic, providing tailored editorial support and steering the book to become its most helpful best.

Index